PREDIABETES WAKE-UP CALL

A Personal Road Map to Prevent Diabetes

Beth Ann Petro Roybal, M.A.

Foreword by
Debbie Nemecek, RN, BSN, CDE

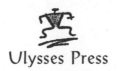

Ulysses Press

Published by: Ulysses Press
P.O. Box 3440
Berkeley, CA 94703
www.ulyssespress.com

Library of Congress Control Number: 2005930012
ISBN: 1-56975-512-4

Printed in Canada by Transcontinental Printing

10 9 8 7 6 5 4 3 2 1

Editor: Mark Woodworth
Editorial and production staff: Kathryn Brooks, Lily Chou, Claire Chun, Nicholas Denton-Brown, Matt Orendorff
Acquisitions Editor: Ashley Chase
Cover Design: Leslie Henriques
Indexer: Sayre Van Young

Distributed by Publishers Group West

This book has been written and published strictly for informational purposes, and in no way should it be used as a substitute for consultation with your medical doctor or health care professional. All facts in this book came from medical files, clinical journals, scientific publications, personal interviews, published trade books, self-published materials by experts, magazine articles, and the personal-practice experiences of the authorities quoted or sources cited. You should not consider educational material herein to be the practice of medicine or to replace consultation with a physician or other medical practitioner. The author and publisher are providing you with information in this work so that you can have the knowledge and can choose, at your own risk, to act on that knowledge. The author and publisher also urge all readers to be aware of their health status and to consult health professionals before beginning any health program, including changes in dietary habits.

To all the diabetes educators and other health professionals who are doing their best to help us stay on the road to better health. Thanks for your dedicaton to our well-being!

TABLE OF CONTENTS

FOREWORD

This book is the first I've ever seen on the complexities that are prediabetes and Syndrome X. It does a wonderful job of making difficult concepts easy to understand and outlines a treatment program that's easy to follow. I plan on using the book for our one-on-one appointments.

I laughed when Beth mentioned that health care providers are too nice to mention the nitty gritty of diabetes complications; she's right and I'm trying to make some changes in that regard. In my years as a diabetes educator in a community hospital, I'm always amazed at what doctors tell their patients (and patients accept) about prediabetes: that their blood sugar is "a little high," which means come back next year. Or if they just lose some weight (without any education on how to do so) they'd be fine.

I love her analogy of the car and the roadtrip—it really makes things fun and understandable. I also like that she uses herself as an example. It's a much more personal approach.

Debbie Nemecek, RN, BSN, CDE
Coordinator of the Outpatient Diabetes Program,
Methodist Hospital
Arcadia, California

INTRODUCTION:
SO THE DOCTOR SAID YOU HAVE "PREDIABETES"...

"My doctor said I have prediabetes. But she didn't really tell me what to do about it." Sound familiar? That's what my friend Jaimie mentioned while we were talking about the type 2 diabetes workbook I had just finished writing. A few days later, I was trying to justify my absence from my son's baseball game. I explained to one of the coaches, Russ, that I was scheduled to discuss diabetes and health writing at a community writers' forum. He backed off immediately, saying, "Hey, you know, my dad has diabetes. My wife and I are both borderline. And I'm worried about my two kids."

It seems that every time someone finds out that I write about diabetes, they have a story or two to share:

"My mom has diabetes..."

"My grandfather had to use insulin..."

"I had diabetes while I was pregnant..."

"My doctor says my sugar is high..."

"I wonder if I'm at risk? I noticed that..."

What's *your* story?

All of us have reason to be concerned. An estimated 17 million people in the United States actually have been diagnosed with type 2 diabetes—that's 1 person in 17. And 20 to 40 million more of us are "borderline"—belonging to that huge category between health and diabetes called "prediabetes." *Epidemic* is not too strong a word to apply to this growing medical crisis. But why do the numbers keep rising? Why is that road to diabetes getting so crowded? Is developing diabetes practically inevitable these days?

I have these questions, too—and not just because I'm a health writer. My mom has diabetes. My aunt died of diabetes-related complications. I'm a few pounds overweight. I'm not as active as I used to be…. Bottom line: I'm definitely at risk. So I was excited when Ulysses Press asked me to write this book about that not-quite-healthy, not-quite-sick condition called "prediabetes." It gives me an opportunity to tell you how type 2 diabetes develops slowly over a long time, how prediabetes can be diagnosed years before diabetes occurs, how you can tell whether you're at risk, and what you can do about it if you are.

I'm not a medical professional. But I do know how to research medical information and present that often-overwhelming medical "techno-talk" at a level you can both understand and use. My goal is to help us help ourselves along the road to better health. For your part, I ask only that you take prediabetes—and the chances of its developing into diabetes—seriously. That's because diabetes can be a nasty disease, going hand-in-hand with heart problems, blood vessel damage, nerve damage, and other serious health problems. You are in the perfect position to do something NOW to prevent or delay all this. As my friend Jane said, "The thing, as you well know, is that most of America either has prediabetes or is heading there. For me, it was a wake-up call." And she didn't even know it was the title to this book!

Use This Book as Your Travel Guide

A prediabetes wake-up call may have gotten *your* attention, too. Now that you've awakened and taken notice, what's next? It's time to get moving…on the road toward a healthier way of life. The route you take to deal with prediabetes is a personal one, based on your own circumstances, preferences, and needs. Use this book to inform yourself about what that road ahead might look like and the many strategies from which you can choose to reach your destination: lower blood glucose levels and better health.

My guess is that you'd rather not have to read this book at all—preferring instead to hit that "snooze" button and go back to sleep, not having to worry about something as uncertain and scary as prediabetes. But, as you'll find out along the course of reading this book, failure to change your direction now can lead to even bigger health problems down the road. I've tried to make reading this book more of a pleasure and less of a chore—I don't like to read stuff like this, either! Here are some features that I hope you'll appreciate and perhaps even enjoy:

- **Conversational language** with true stories and personal examples
- **Travel talk** to describe how prediabetes and diabetes develop and how you can head back toward a healthier destination
- **Stop & Think!** boxes contain powerful statistics about prediabetes and diabetes

- **Buzzwords** likely to spew from the mouths of your health care providers, <u>underlined</u> in the text and defined more fully in the "Learning the Buzz" section at the end of the book
- **Support Team** boxes provide suggestions on how your road crew—the people in your life—can better support your choices for better health
- **Questions for Consideration** at the end of each chapter, to help you reflect on what the information might mean for your travel toward health

Once you have made it through this travel guide, feel free to share your thoughts—especially what helped and what didn't—as well as stories from your own prediabetes journey. Send any feedback or comments to me in care of Ulysses Press, P.O. Box 3440, Berkeley, CA 94703. They'll be sure I get it. Or reach me more directly through my website: www.bethroybal.com.

Wishing you happy, healthy travels,

Beth

PART I

PART I

From "Pre" to "D"—A Slow,
Winding, Bumpy Road

Think about good health, prediabetes, and diabetes as if they were different sections of the same road. You may have started off healthy enough, cruising along through your life's journey enjoying the view. But over the years, small, almost unnoticeable problems arose: gaining a little extra weight, not watching what you eat, becoming less active, dealing with other health concerns, taking care of everyone but yourself…. Then one day, you reach a sign that says:

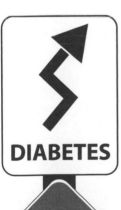

The sign is so big, it's hard to ignore. And so are the bumps, potholes, cracks, and other obstacles in the road that you've been noticing. But the warning might still be surprising to you. How in the world did you get to such a place, anyway?

Actually, the goal is for you NOT to get there—to find a way back toward the smooth road and good health. I'll start by giving you an idea of how that road got so rough in the first place, how prediabetes and diabetes occur. The short story is that prediabetes and diabetes are conditions that result when your body can't properly digest and use the food you eat. The levels of sugar in your blood remain consistently too high. The full version is a bit more complex. It'll take us about three chapters to explain the basics:

Chapter 1 describes how your body digests and uses food.

Chapter 2 shows how the process of using food for fuel can go wrong, leading to prediabetes and diabetes.

Chapter 3 explains why you should care—what diabetes might mean in your daily life and to your overall health.

1

HOW FOOD FUELS YOUR BODY

To take a long journey, you need a reliable vehicle. But that's not all: The vehicle needs something to propel itself with—an engine. For a car, plane, or train, that engine takes the form of a motor. For a bike, rowboat, or skateboard, that engine is *you*. What makes the engines work? Fuel. What kind of fuel? Food.

The starting point for understanding how good health can turn into prediabetes and eventually even type 2 diabetes is to know how your body digests and uses the food you eat to make the fuel that powers you along, like the way your car's motor turns gasoline into motion. The process is quite incredible, when you stop to think about it: You're hungry. You grab something to eat, take a bite, chew, and swallow. Down it goes, into that dark, dank world known as your digestive system. Somehow, your body finds a way to use or store most of that food. The waste? Well, you know that end of the story....

The first question is this: What's so important about the food you eat? And then, what happens to get food from your mouth to where the nutrients are needed? Let's answer these questions in turn.

Food, Glorious Fuel

Whatever its taste, texture, or amount, all food is made up of various combinations of similar components: carbohydrates, proteins, fats, and vitamins and minerals. Food may contain other parts, too, such as alcohol and other substances that have yet to be discovered. Let's take a closer look at the groups of nutrients to see how your body uses them.

Carbohydrates for Fuel

Believe it or not, *every* cell of your body uses <u>carbohydrates</u>. Even more: Every cell of your body *needs* carbohydrates. These carbon-containing substances originate from plants. And plants rely on photosynthesis, the unique process of using light to help create energy—specifically, to change carbon dioxide and water into carbohydrates.

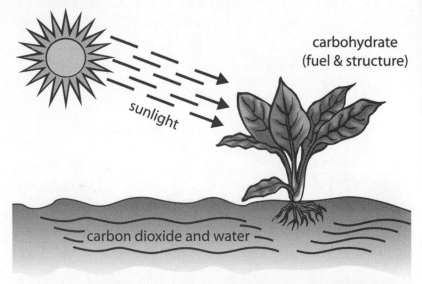

carbohydrate
(fuel & structure)

sunlight

carbon dioxide and water

Carbs provide the energy for plants—and eventually for us humans, as well. Carbohydrates also help plants maintain their structures, serving as the equivalent of an animal's skeleton or shell. Carbohydrates are divided into several groups, usually classified as sugars, starches, cellulose, and gums. We'll simplify this to three: sugar, starch, and fiber.

What are all these carbs good for? In the plant world, <u>sugars</u> are the fuels that plants "burn" directly for energy. <u>Starches</u> are stored fuel, waiting patiently in certain plant cells until they're needed, at which time they, too, are broken down into sugars. <u>Fiber</u> is the stringy, chunky, bark-like stuff that keeps plants from flopping over and helps them retain moisture.

One day, a plant is harvested and turned into food for people. Some plants are used raw, like lettuce. Others are processed a bit, like rolled oats—or a lot, like finely milled and bleached wheat flour, which may then be used in a variety of baked goods.

You take a bite of that food. Chewing and mixing the food with saliva makes it break down a bit. But the real work begins once food hits your stomach and then travels through the rest of your digestive tract. Most of the carbs, especially the sugars and some starches, are broken down into fuel for your cells to use. Some are broken down quickly, others more slowly, depending on their particles' size and complexity. The most common form of carb-based fuel is <u>glucose</u>.

Here's what you need to remember about all this:

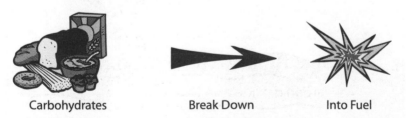

Carbohydrates   Break Down   Into Fuel

And that fuel is called glucose. You're going to hear this word *a lot*, both in this book and out there in your "real world"—especially at doctor's appointments and such.

Starches and fiber help regulate the sugar-breakdown process. Starches, remember, are *stored* forms of carbohydrates. So they can be changed into fuel, but more slowly than sugars.

This helps keep your body from having to deal with too much sugar hitting the bloodstream all at once. It's sort of like the propane tank in my side yard: A truck comes periodically to fill up the tank with liquified propane. My tank stores the fuel, and releases it as a gas when needed to heat up water or run the furnace.

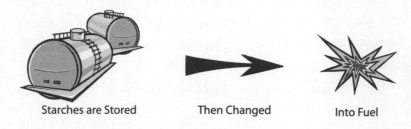

Starches are Stored   Then Changed   Into Fuel

Fiber helps control the speed of digestion, not only of carbo-hydrates but also of the other components of food. Some kinds of fiber help control appetite as well, absorbing liquid to make you feel full.

This chart below sums up the types of carbs in your food, as well as what they do inside your body.

Type of Carb	Food Sources	How It's Used
Sugar	Fruits, vegetables, milk, table sugar	Broken down into glucose to provide fuel for the body's cells
Starch	Grains, legumes (beans and peas), potatoes, seed	Some is broken down into glucose to provide fuel for the body's cells; the rest is stored for later use.
Fiber	Fruits, grains, legumes, vegetables	Regulates the speed at which other nutrients are absorbed.

Fats for Fuel and Protection

Fat and fat-like substances are found throughout the body and in much of the food you eat. Your body digests it all, turning some of the digested fat into fuel, while using other digested fat for protection: insulating your body from cold, cushioning important organs, and performing other functions. One of the fat-like substances, cholesterol, helps waterproof your skin, line your nerves, and carry fat around in your blood vessels.

If you've eaten more than your body can use, the body doesn't get rid of the excess. Instead, extra fat circulates through your blood until it can be stored. Fat storage cells are—well, you know where to find them—around your abdomen, hips, thighs, and other places throughout your body.

This chart sums up the kinds of fats you find in the food you eat and their common sources.

Type of Fat	Food Sources
Saturated	Meat, coconut and palm oil, high-fat dairy products
Trans	Partially hydrogenated oils, hydrogenated shortening used in baked goods, fast foods
Polyunsaturated	Fish, vegetable oils, nuts, seeds
Monounsaturated	Vegetables and vegetable oils, nuts, seeds
Cholesterol (fat-like substance)	Egg yolks, shellfish, meat, dairy products

Protein for Power

Protein is used to build muscle and other tissue, as well as to make hormones and other substances needed by the body. Once you eat a bite of protein, your body disassembles it into various amino acids, then recombines them into the specific amino acids it needs. The following chart summarizes the sources of protein and how they're used.

Food Sources of Protein	How They're Used
Meat, poultry, seafood, eggs, dairy, legumes, grains, seeds	Build muscle and other tissue, are changed into hormones to help various bodily processes

Vitamins and Minerals

Vitamins and minerals aren't consumed for fuel—and vitamins aren't even incorporated into body cells. So what makes vitamins and minerals so important to your health?

Vitamins are made up of various combinations of the chemicals carbon, oxygen, hydrogen, and nitrogen. They serve as the assistants, or *catalysts*, for all your body's functions. For instance, some vitamins help the cells burn glucose, fat, and protein for fuel. Others help build bone (vitamin D) or repair damaged arteries (vitamins C and E). The list of vitamins—and their roles—is long, and getting longer each year as more vitamin-like substances are discovered.

Minerals are substances that occur naturally in rocks and soil. Iron, zinc, copper, and calcium are a few examples. Plants take up dissolved minerals when they absorb water from the ground. Animals receive minerals from eating plants—or from eating other animals that have already absorbed minerals from plants. Your body uses minerals to assist in a range of functions, from thinking to maintaining your heartbeat. Some minerals are used to form parts of your body: Calcium is a component of bone, for example. Altogether your body uses more than 20 different minerals.

Other Components of Food

A myriad of other food components exist, but don't necessarily fit into one of the main categories we've already talked about. Alcohol, for example, is similar to carbohydrates; however, your

THE DIGESTIVE SYSTEM

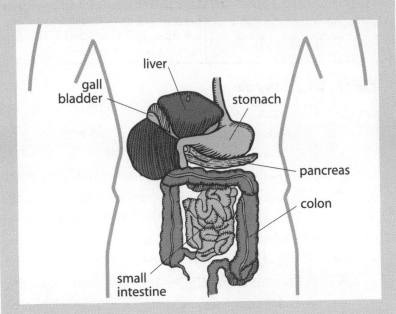

Stomach: A large sac that begins breaking food down, sending the smaller particles into the intestines.

Small intestine: This long, coiled-up tube continues breaking down food into smaller and smaller pieces, allowing tiny particles to pass through the side wall into the bloodstream.

Colon: This larger, "question mark"–shaped tube receives particles that can't be used and allows water to flow from the waste through its walls into the bloodstream. The end of the colon, the rectum, is where waste leaves your body.

Gallbladder: A small sac that stores digestive juices (bile) and sends the juices to the stomach.

Liver: The body's main chemical factory, making bile for digestion as well as other chemicals needed by the body.

Pancreas: Another chemical factory, creating both digestive juices for the intestines and insulin to carry fuel from the bloodstream into your cells.

body breaks down alcohol somewhat differently than it does carbs. Alcohol also contains more calories than do carbs. Other food components are being discovered all the time. Ask a dietitian to give you the latest list!

Creating Fuel from Food

Now you know food is made up of a range of nutrients, used for fuel and various other functions inside your body. But how does that food change from a bite of burger to a molecule of fuel? And what does all this have to do with prediabetes and diabetes?

That's where the whole process of <u>digestion</u> comes in. You probably know about the stomach and its role. Meet some other players in the digestive process:

1. Your stomach gets busy mashing the food this way and that, mixing it with digestive juices sent by the gallbladder. These acids begin to break the food down into smaller particles.

2. The smaller pieces of food travel from the stomach into the small intestine, where more digestive enzymes from the pancreas break the food down into even smaller pieces. The smallest particles are absorbed through the walls of the small intestine and pass into your bloodstream.

3. Special chemicals (hormones) made by the pancreas and liver lead the food particles to where they're needed. One of these hormones is insulin, made in the pancreas.

4. Fat goes toward lining nerves, cushioning organs, and other uses. Some is turned into fuel for the cells. The rest keeps circulating in the bloodstream or is stored in cells for later use.

5. Protein pieces (amino acids) are recombined into muscle tissue and hormones. These protein-based helpers, as well

as other food components such as vitamins and minerals, aid body processes.

6. Carbohydrates are broken into smaller packages of sugar, called glucose. Glucose molecules are led into each cell, where they're used to produce energy. Any extra glucose continues to roam the bloodstream until it can be used or pulled out of the blood by the kidneys. Insulin made by the pancreas is the hormone responsible for finding glucose and getting it into the cells.

We've taken the process up to the time when the food is absorbed into your bloodstream. What's next? The various nutrients speed through the bloodstream to where they're needed. How do they know where to go? How do they get inside the cells? That's the next part of the story.

Insulin: The Glucose Helper

Glucose and other nutrients can't simply leap from blood vessels into cells. They need some help. That's where insulin comes to the rescue. You might hear insulin referred to as the "key" that unlocks the "door" to the cell. Using our travel analogy, perhaps you can think of insulin as a fuel additive that makes the fuel burn better. Here's how the process works: When you eat, the body signals your pancreas to crank out insulin. Insulin pours into the bloodstream and searches for glucose. It hooks on, then leads glucose into the cells. As you might guess, this routine ramps up for a few hours after you eat, then slows down after most of the glucose is put where it needs to end up. So you naturally have changing levels of glucose and insulin throughout the day, to match your body's need—higher levels of both right after a meal, lower levels of both right before your next meal. If your pancreas makes enough insulin to deal with the glucose, then everything's great. Insulin leads the glucose into the cells, the cells burn their fuel, and your body functions well. Your body is working like a finely tuned race car.

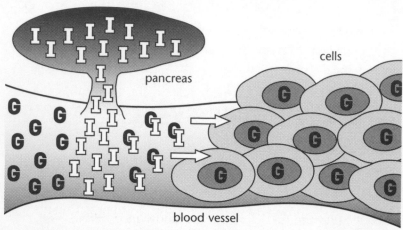

Insulin/Glucose Balance

But what happens if there isn't enough insulin? Or there's too much glucose? In the next chapter we'll talk about what can go wrong with this process, and why.

Questions for Consideration

- What's the primary role of carbohydrates in your body?
- What part does insulin play in the use of food for fuel?
- How might this information about nutrients and digestion fit—or not fit—with any diet or eating plan you're following these days?

2

WHEN THE FUEL SYSTEM
BREAKS DOWN

After reading the first chapter, you know more about food and the normal digestive process. You have a pretty good idea of the nutrients contained in food. You've learned how your body breaks food down and absorbs its nutrients into your bloodstream. And you found out that the pancreas makes a special chemical called insulin that leads glucose from the bloodstream into each cell. Remember, though, we left off with two questions:

- What happens if there isn't enough insulin to carry glucose into the cells?
- What if there's too much glucose in the bloodstream?

I promised to give you an answer. Here it is, short and not-so-sweet:

Diabetes

I'll use the rest of this chapter to explain the details. Just as I relied on the analogy of the road to describe how prediabetes and diabetes develop, I'll use the concept of a car's fuel system to explain more about the problems that can arise with glucose.

Fuel Floods the System

What's your favorite car to drive? I love my butter-colored 1988 Honda Civic, all 290,000 miles of it. When I start it up in the morning, the engine purrs. I get to shift it through all five speeds as I negotiate the turns and hills and potholes on the way to taking my kids to school. And despite its age, the Civic still gets almost 40 miles per gallon of gasoline. Recently, though, a problem arose. Whenever I stopped the car out in the sun, it wouldn't restart. If I waited a few minutes, then it would finally start up and run fine for the rest of the trip. For several months, I simply put up with it. But the next time I had to have the car tested for emissions to renew the registration, it failed miserably. Time to get a new car? Fortunately, no. My favorite car guy, Dave, and his staff determined the cause: the fuel sensor, which had been slowly losing its ability to maintain the optimal oxygen–fuel mix. After they replaced the sensor, the car passed the smog test easily. And it's back on the road again, purring like a kitten.

That's sort of what it's like with the fuel glucose and <u>diabetes</u>. Remember from the last chapter that once glucose enters the blood, insulin needs to lead glucose into the cells. But sometimes the fuel—in this case, the glucose—backs up in the bloodstream rather than entering into the cells. A snapshot of your blood vessels might look something like the diagram on page 23.

Compared to the snapshot in the previous chapter, your "fuel lines" are becoming flooded with glucose. Your body may not be difficult to start in sunny weather like my Civic, but consistently high levels of glucose in your blood can cause other problems:

- The cells don't get the fuel they need. They're starving! You may feel rundown and irritable, lose weight, and have other symptoms.
- The body—especially the pancreas and <u>kidneys</u>—gets tired of having to deal with all the extra glucose. Over

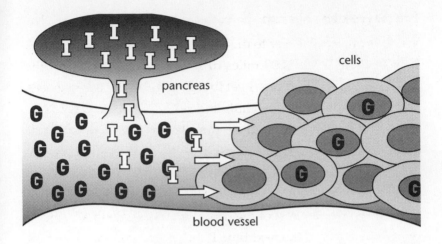

Too Much Glucose in Bloodstream

time, the pancreas may slow down its work of making insulin. Then the kidneys can't handle the extra workload of filtering out the extra glucose.

- The extra glucose in the blood can damage the blood vessels themselves, affecting your heart, your eyes, your nerves, your gums, your feet, your reproductive organs (yikes!), and more.

You might wonder: "What causes glucose to build up?" or maybe even "Why can't my insulin handle the job?" Let's take a look at a couple of ways these things can happen.

When the Pancreas Stops Making Insulin: Type 1 Diabetes

In some people, the pancreas simply stops making insulin. It usually happens rather suddenly. Often, this form of diabetes—called type 1 diabetes—occurs after the body attacks the pancreas, mistaking it for a virus, bacterium, or other dangerous threat. Type 1 diabetes also occurs when the pancreas is removed, as a result of injury, cancer, or other health problem.

You may also have heard type 1 referred to as insulin-dependent diabetes or juvenile diabetes. Some 5 to 10 percent of people with diabetes have type 1.

Without insulin, glucose quickly builds up in the blood. The cells starve. The body begins to burn fat for fuel, creating toxins. The kidneys become overloaded with glucose and toxins. Without added insulin, death would result. Because the pancreas makes no insulin, people with type 1 must inject insulin to survive.

The good news for you is that prediabetes does *not* lead to type 1 diabetes. So we won't discuss this type of diabetes further.

When Insulin Doesn't Get the Job Done: Type 2 Diabetes

Sometimes glucose builds up in the bloodstream even when insulin *is* present. This is called type 2 diabetes. You may also have heard it called non-insulin-dependent diabetes mellitus (NIDDM) or adult onset diabetes. Roughly 90 to 95 percent of people with diabetes have this type—about 17 million people in the United States, for example. Sadly, adults aren't the only ones dealing with type 2 diabetes anymore. Many young children and teens are also developing this disease. And many people of all ages are heading toward type 2 diabetes, falling into that strange category called prediabetes. Sound familiar? But how does type 2 happen? Let's take another look at my car.

Just like the way the fuel sensor on my car gradually gave out before I noticed a real problem, type 2 diabetes develops slowly over the course of many years. The process often begins when the body's cells can't use insulin properly. This might occur as a result of one or more of these factors:

- A tendency toward diabetes passed down from your parents or grandparents
- Excess weight

- Being physically inactive
- Immune system disorders such as lupus
- Feeling high levels of stress for a long time
- Taking certain medications such as steroids
- Overexposure to toxins (endocrine disruptors) such as fertilizers or pesticides
- Having had gestational diabetes (GDM) (that is, diabetes that develops while you're pregnant but usually goes away after you give birth)

The body responds to these or other challenges by making extra chemicals that keep it from using insulin. You'll hear this called insulin resistance. There *is* insulin present—it just can't work the way it needs to.

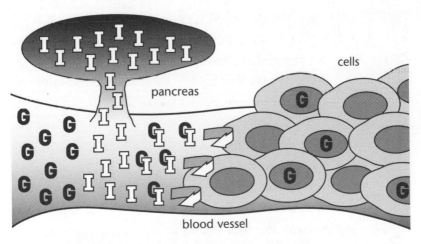

Insulin Resistance: Insulin Doesn't Work Right

In other cases, the pancreas makes too little insulin to deal with the glucose load. This might be caused by a problem with the pancreas, or by a person consistently eating more food (which converts to glucose) than their body can handle. The bloodstream might look something like this:

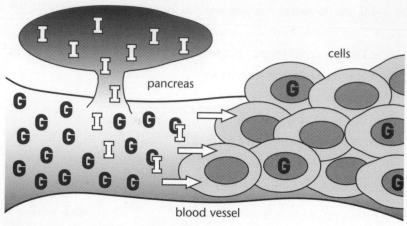

Pancreas Makes too Little Insulin

Most people with type 2 diabetes have some combination of insulin resistance *and* glucose–insulin imbalance at the same time. Here's one way this can happen: Insulin made by the pancreas is not effective in leading glucose into the cells. Over time, the pancreas may start to give up. It makes less and less

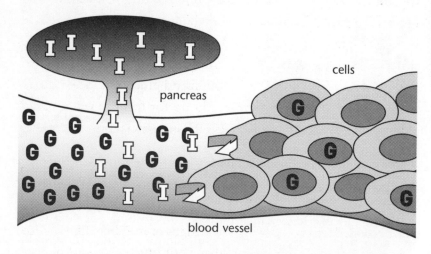

Insulin Resistance and Glucose-Insulin Imbalance

insulin—not enough to get the job done. The lack of insulin allows glucose to build up even more in the bloodstream.

Let's use another graphic to sum up conceptually how type 2 diabetes occurs in most people:

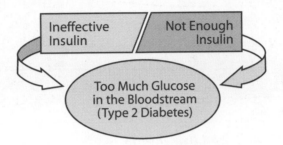

But What about Prediabetes?

You would think that either you have type 2 diabetes...or you don't. At one level, that's true. But like many ongoing (<u>chronic</u>) health problems, type 2 diabetes usually develops slowly over the course of many years. That's how "they" (you know, the medical experts) came up with a whole category called prediabetes. It's likely you might not even notice symptoms of the condition for a long time. Still, inside your body, changes in how your body produces and uses insulin and glucose may be occurring. These changes are setting you up for future trouble. This transitional phase—our road with the occasional bump in it—is what is referred to as "prediabetes."

By the Numbers

Maybe it'll help to take a look at how glucose is measured in your blood. Then you can see the ranges of numbers that health care pros use to determine whether your glucose levels are normal, impaired (prediabetes), or high (diabetes).

First, you'll need to remember that the amount of glucose found in your blood varies throughout the day. Levels tend to be lower before meals, since you haven't eaten anything for a while. Levels tend to be higher after meals, as the food you've eaten is digested and the resulting glucose enters your bloodstream on its way to the cells. For people who don't have diabetes or prediabetes, daily glucose ranges might look something like this:

Time	Normal Blood Glucose Levels
Before meals	80-100 mg/dL
1–2 hours after meals	100–140 mg/dL
After a large evening meal	Up to 180 mg/dL

You'll notice the metric abbreviations "mg/dL" after the numbers. This means "milligrams of glucose per deciliter of blood." It's the standard measurement used in most blood glucose tests.

Several lab tests can be done to measure blood glucose levels. Some are done right in your doctor's office, while others are performed at a laboratory. These tests give you an overall picture of your glucose levels. The most common tests used to diagnosis prediabetes and diabetes are the fasting glucose test and the glucose challenge test (GCT). Here's more information about each.

Fasting Glucose Test

In this test, blood is drawn and tested after you've gone without food or drink for at least 8 hours. This gives you an idea of how well your body uses glucose when food isn't readily available. The fasting glucose test is usually the preferred test for diagnosing whether you have prediabetes or diabetes.

Fasting Glucose Test Ranges	
Normal	Less than 100 mg/dL
Impaired (prediabetes)	100–125 mg/dL
High (diabetes)	126 mg/dL or higher

Glucose Challenge Test

This test may be done right after a fasting test, or it may be done separately. You drink a glucose mixture, then wait for 1 or 2 hours. Blood is then drawn and your glucose level measured.

Glucose Challenge Test Ranges (Ranges are the same for both 1 hour and 2 hours)	
Normal	Less than 140 mg/dL
Impaired (prediabetes)	140–199 mg/dL
High (diabetes)	200 mg/dL or greater

The Diagnosis of Prediabetes— What Does It Mean?

If your numbers come within the impaired range of either test, your doctor may decide that you do have prediabetes. This means that for some reason, too much glucose is floating around in your bloodstream. It may be because your body doesn't make enough insulin, you eat more food for fuel than you can handle, for some reason your insulin isn't working right, or a combination of all these factors. But what's the big deal? Why should you worry? After all, you haven't been diagnosed with diabetes…yet. The next chapter takes a look at some of these questions you might have.

Questions for Consideration

- If your doctor has said you have prediabetes, do you know why they arrived at that diagnosis?
- Do you know your blood glucose test results? If so, what are they?
- Do you have a plan for monitoring your glucose periodically to make sure your levels are not rising even higher?

3

WHY WORRY ABOUT IT?

This is the chapter where I want to scare you half to death—not to be mean, but to help you realize the seriousness of prediabetes and the potential implications if you do nothing to get off the diabetes road. Are my tactics fair? Maybe not. But neither is type 2 diabetes. Don't just take my word for it. Read these stories and facts to get the real picture. Then move on to Part II to learn more about your risk, and then to Part III to find out more about your routes back to better health.

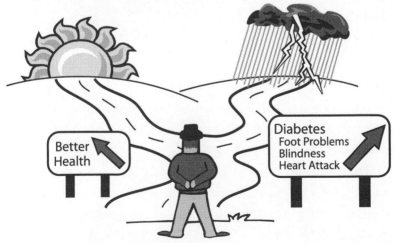

The Grim Truth about Diabetes

There's no way around it: Diabetes can be a horrible disease. Health care professionals are generally kind people and refrain from scare tactics; but you need to know what you're possibly up against so that you can do something now to avoid it. Here's what happened to Bob, for example, my brother-in-law's brother-in-law (just so you know I'm not making this up!). He was a big man—both in size and in importance as a high-level manager at a company just outside Chicago. After years of running the plant, it was time to slow down, retire, and spend some fun time with his children and grandchildren. Instead, Bob spent his free time—when he wasn't enduring four hours of kidney dialysis four days a week—beside his backyard pool in Florida, in a wheelchair, one foot amputated, still smoking a pack or two of cigarettes a day. Bob died in the hospital from complications related to type 2 diabetes, after having his other foot amputated. His 30-something daughter had dropped dead of a heart attack a year earlier, after failing to follow her own plan to manage diabetes (she had type 1 diabetes).

There's Good News, Too

"My father, who is almost 87 years of age, decided to lose weight, and he takes no medication. He has had diabetes for more than 20 years with no complications." That's the story of another person who is also dealing with type 2 diabetes. She is doing all she can, too, to manage her diabetes so that she can remain as active as her father.

Then, there's my mom. She has had diabetes for many years but has been taking her meds, watching her diet, and getting regular exercise. She's remained reasonably healthy and active. She feels some aches and pains and experiences other bothersome health problems such as high blood pressure and arthritis, but not so different than the rest of the folks her age. Now in her 70s, she's enjoying life, taking care of the grandkids, volunteering at church, traveling around the country with my dad, visiting me regularly in California, and making crafts to sell at Christmas shows. All in all, not a bad life!

Your Prediabetes Crossroad

Many folks don't take the threat of prediabetes or even diabetes very seriously. As my friend Jane learned, "A lot of people—and especially doctors—pooh-pooh the diabetes thing. When I mention it, even to my primary doctor, he starts telling me I'm too hung up on 'titles.'" Yet the evidence continues to grow that people with diabetes who manage it well lessen their chances of complications. And people with prediabetes who manage it well are less likely to go on to develop diabetes. So one lesson here is that the quicker you turn back toward health from the prediabetes road, the more likely it is you'll remain reasonably well and relatively complication-free. As in all things in life, you have a choice:

- To possibly end up like Bob by ignoring the warning signs or
- To work toward maintaining good health and enjoying your life, like my friend Jane, my mother, and that 87-year-old man, who all took consistent steps to manage their diabetes and maintain their health

What route will *you* choose? Just to be sure you know what the consequences of inaction can be, let's review some of diabetes's common complications.

The Complications of Diabetes

Complications refers to health problems that have been linked to a particular disease. In this case, *many* health conditions have been linked to diabetes. This means that people with diabetes are more likely to have these problems. Take a look at the list. It's a long one. My goal is not to depress you, but rather to help you realize that you are in a position *now*—while you're still in the "prediabetes" diagnosis category—to do something to prevent or delay these health problems.

Cardiovascular Problems. *Cardio-* means "heart" and *vascular* means "blood vessels." Heart and blood vessel problems go together like a horse and carriage. That's because the heart is the "machine" that pumps blood through the vessels. A problem anywhere in the system damages how the whole system works.

If you've been given the diagnosis of "prediabetes," then you are *already* at risk of having <u>cardiovascular problems</u>. If you progress on to diabetes, your risk grows even greater. Why the link? It's not totally understood. But what *is* known is that the same hormone, insulin, that leads glucose into cells for fuel also helps lead fat into other cells for storage. If you lack enough insulin or if it doesn't work right, the fat continues to circulate in your bloodstream. With too much fat *and* too much glucose floating around, it's no wonder the vessels get clogged. The net result? Raising your blood pressure, creating clots, and putting extra strain on your heart. Heart attack and stroke are probably two cardiovascular problems you already know about. But there are more: kidney failure, circulation problems, vision loss, problems with healing, and more. We'll talk about these later.

 Of every six people who have diabetes, four of them will die from heart problems. The saddest part is that probably three of the four could have lived longer, had they taken steps toward heart health.

Foot Problems. Even in the healthiest person, the body has to work harder to send blood high up in the body, the heart, to the far ends: the feet. Add in nerve and blood vessel damage caused by diabetes, and perhaps high blood pressure or high blood-fat levels as well, and it's no wonder that people with diabetes commonly have foot ailments. Here are some typical ones:

- Nail fungus
- Bone spurs and other bony growths
- Lack of sensation in the feet (neuropathy)
- Slow healing, which can eventually lead to gangrene and foot amputation
- Foot pain

Eye Problems. Many folks with high glucose levels notice blurry vision. This often clears up when glucose levels come down to normal ranges. More serious eye problems result from having high glucose levels for many years. Each of these can result in vision loss or in blindness:

- Cataracts (clouding of the lenses of the eyes)
- Glaucoma (fluid build-up and high pressure inside the eye)
- Retinopathy (damaged, leaky blood vessels in the back of the eye)

 More than 6 out of 10 people with type 2 diabetes show signs of retinopathy within the first 20 years of being diagnosed.

Nerve Problems (Neuropathy). No one's really sure yet why high blood glucose levels lead to nerve problems. But the longer a person has diabetes, the more likely it is that they'll develop neuropathy. Nerves are found throughout the body, carrying control signals from the brain to the rest of the body and returning information from parts of the body back to the brain. So people with diabetes may experience nerve-related problems anywhere in the body. Common problems are lack of sensation or feelings of pain or tingling. Systems that are controlled by nerves, such as digestion, may also be affected. A condition called gastroparesis can be due to neuropathy, resulting in severe nausea, pain, and diarrhea.

Kidney Disease (<u>Nephropathy</u>). The body's two kidneys normally remove toxins from the blood, sending them out through urine. If they have to work too hard for a long time, as occurs with consistently high glucose levels, the kidneys slowly lose the ability to filter toxins properly. Instead, they let other valuable substances such as protein leak out. Plus, kidneys in a body with diabetes have a lot more toxins to filter out than do kidneys in a normal body. If this situation continues over time, the kidneys begin to give up. Not only do they allow toxins to build up and protein to leak out, but the owner of the body ends up feeling tired all the time. This condition is referred to as End-stage Renal Disease (ESRD). Kidney dialysis is an attempt to help do what the kidneys no longer can: filter toxins from the blood. Transplant of a kidney from a donor is another potential option to restore some kidney function.

 In the United States and Europe, the most common cause of end-stage renal (kidney) disease is diabetes. Especially hard hit in the United States are Native Americans, Hispanics (particularly Mexican Americans), and African Americans.

Dental Problems. The changes diabetes makes to blood vessels can also make gum disease more likely. <u>Gingivitis</u> is the term dentists use for inflamed gums. <u>Periodontitis</u> is the next stage, when the gums pull away from your teeth. The resulting pockets can become infected with bacteria, which thrive on the high levels of glucose in your blood. This leads to tooth decay and loss, with consequent eating and nutrition problems.

Pregnancy Problems. Having diabetes and being pregnant can lead to problems. Often, any existing complications such as eye problems become worse during pregnancy. Retinopathy, high blood pressure, or thyroid problems may also occur for the first time during pregnancy. The greatest risk for women with type 2 diabetes is having large babies. Miscarriages and stillbirths also happen more frequently in women with diabetes than in the rest of the female population. And babies born to women with uncontrolled diabetes are at much greater risk for having major birth defects. Many of these defects occur in the earliest stages of pregnancy—before you may know you're pregnant.

Other Health Problems. People with diabetes are at greater risk for other health problems too. These can range from the flu and pneumonia to other immune system problems such as some types of arthritis. Recent research has even uncovered a possible connection between diabetes and Alzheimer's disease.

Don't Panic—Take Action!

Time to stop and take a breath. Remember, you're not in the diabetes category...yet. You *can* do something to help prevent or delay type 2 diabetes and its associated complications. The time to start, though, is right now, today. And the rest of this book will give you suggestions for how to get going on the road back to health.

Questions for Consideration

- Do you know of anyone in your family or circle of friends who has had to deal with complications associated with diabetes?
- Which potential complications scare you most?
- Have you noticed any health problems already that might be related to diabetes? If so, are you seeking treatment for them?

PART II

How Did You End Up on Prediabetes Street? All about Risk Factors

Have you ever headed off on a trip, sure of where you're going, only to find yourself lost and confused? Nothing looks familiar, you have no idea where you are, and you certainly don't know which is the right road to take to your destination.

"Where in the heck am I—and how did I get here?"

Take a look around you. Like it or not, you're in Prediabetes Land. You've received a diagnosis of prediabetes, probably because your blood glucose levels were consistently higher than "normal," but not yet high enough to earn the dubious "diabetes" distinction. How did you get here? How are you going to find your way out of this mess?

Just like getting lost on a road trip, your first step in dealing with prediabetes is to stop right where you are. Take a breath. Get your bearings. That's what Part II is all about. We'll take a close look at the underlying factors that nudged you onto this prediabetes road. By understanding how you got to this point, you'll be better able to find your way back onto a smoother path, rather than finding yourself going around in endless circles or—even worse—heading the wrong way onto Diabetes Boulevard.

Risk factors are those things that lead to the development of prediabetes and continue to make you more likely than the average Jane or Joe to develop type 2 diabetes. For some risks, researchers know why they may lead to diabetes. For other risks, they're not so sure. Yet for all risks, researchers *do* know that there's a link between the particular risk and diabetes. Let's divide risk factors into four groups, then take a closer look at each. Here's what we'll be talking about:

- **Speed Bumps:** Aspects of your health, such as having immune system problems or taking certain medications, that increase your risk of developing diabetes
- **Dangerous Curves:** Details of your daily life, such as how much stress you have or what you eat, that increase your risk
- **Unforeseen Mechanical Breakdowns:** "Just because" risks such as your family's health history, your ethnic background, your age, or other things you might not be able to do much about, but that still are linked to diabetes
- **The Diabetes–Cardiovascular Cutoff:** A special group of risks called "Syndrome X" or "metabolic syndrome" that puts you in danger of developing both diabetes and cardiovascular problems

For each set of risk factors, I'll explain what they are and how they may contribute to prediabetes and diabetes. You'll have a chance to assess your own life to determine whether you have any of these risks. Once you've identified your risks, then you'll find it easier to understand and select strategies that can help you get back on the road to better health. That's where Part III takes over.

4

SPEED BUMPS—
YOUR HEALTH RISKS

Don't you hate them? Those speed bumps that force you to slow down, usually when you're in a hurry. As far as your risk for diabetes is concerned, certain health factors can make it more likely that you're facing diabetes up ahead. I'll describe the risks. Then you can check off all that apply to you. The more risks you have, the greater your chances of going on to develop diabetes—and the more pressing your need to take a different direction in your road toward better health.

Speed Bump #1: Having Glucose Intolerance

Glucose intolerance simply means that your body, for some reason, can't seem to deal with all the glucose that is broken down from the food you eat. Glucose intolerance can be caused by a couple of factors:

- **Your body doesn't make enough insulin** to deal with all the glucose in your system, either because there's something wrong with the chemical-making process (see the description in the previous chapter) or because you eat more food than your body needs.

- **The insulin your body makes doesn't work as it should**—it's unable to lead glucose into the cells.

If you want to know more about these problems, go back to Chapter 3 for a quick review.

Glucose intolerance is determined by checking for how much glucose is in your bloodstream. Remember those blood tests we talked about in Chapter 2? The same tests are typically used to decide whether you have glucose intolerance. Here's a summary of the test ranges. I've left space at the bottom for you to fill in your own numbers, if you know them.

COMMON BLOOD GLUCOSE TEST RESULTS

The numbers in the middle "impaired" row are what doctors use to classify you as having prediabetes. All it takes to qualify is *either* an <u>impaired fasting glucose (IFG)</u> result *or* an <u>impaired glucose challenge (IGT)</u> result. Some people have both an IFT *and* an IGT result. No doubt about their diagnosis! Let's say that, in your case, the good news from your results is that the amount of glucose in your blood isn't high enough to earn entry into the "diabetes club." But it's higher than it should be. Something seems to be keeping your body from properly using the glucose in your blood.

	Fasting Glucose Test	Glucose Challenge Test
Normal range	Less than 100 mb/dL	Less than 140 mb/dL
Impaired (prediabetes)	**100-125 mg/dL**	**140-199 mg/dL**
High (possibly diabetes)	126 mg/dL or higher	200 mg/dL or higher
YOUR RESULTS		

Now check the items that apply to you.

Do you eat more food than your body needs?

❑ Yes   ❑ No   ❑ I don't know

Does your body make enough insulin to handle all the glucose in your system?

❑ Yes   ❑ No   ❑ I don't know

Does the insulin in your body work properly to get glucose into the cells?

❑ Yes   ❑ No   ❑ I don't know

Do you have blood glucose test results in the "impaired" range?

❑ Yes   ❑ No   ❑ I don't know

If you answer "yes" to ANY of these questions, then "glucose intolerance" is a risk factor for you. If you answered "no" to ALL these questions, then your doctor has come up with the prediabetes diagnosis based on other risk factors (keep reading!). If you answered "I don't know" to ANY of these questions, check with your doctor the next time you're in for a visit.

Speed Bump #2: Existing Immune System Problems

The immune system is your body's amazing way of fending off threats to your health. Involving several organs and many specialized cells, your immune system routinely handles everything from sending germ-killing cells to help heal a scrape on your knee to using specialized chemicals (hormones) to catch and remove foreign substances such as pollen or dust. All you might notice is a red, bleeding scrape on your knee, or a stuffy nose.

What, you might be wondering, does all this immune system stuff have to do with diabetes? The more researchers learn about diabetes, the more they realize that it may, too, be linked to the immune system. Take type 1 diabetes, for example. Researchers discovered over time that some children develop type 1 (remember, in type 1 diabetes, the pancreas stops making insulin) shortly after having a routine viral infection, such as the flu. For some reason, the immune system gets confused and seems to regard the pancreas as a "foreign" invader, which of course it's not. The immune system mounts an attack against the pancreas, disabling it. And without a functioning pancreas, there's no insulin production.

Type 2 diabetes may not be the direct result of the immune system's attacking the pancreas, yet researchers have noted that people with type 2 diabetes often have immune system problems. Problems of this kind include the following health conditions:

- **Hormone problems:** The chemical messengers made in special organs throughout the body, such as the thyroid, liver, and pancreas, don't work properly or aren't made in great enough quantities.
- **Rheumatoid arthritis:** The body confuses the connective tissue (such as the tissues that hold your joints together) as "foreign" and attacks it, leading to inflammation, destruction of the tissue, and difficulty with movement.
- **Hepatitis C:** People with type 2 diabetes are twice as likely as the rest of the population to have hepatitis C, a chronic disease in which a virus attacks the liver.

There's even some evidence linking diabetes and problems such as Alzheimer's disease. Which came first, the diabetes or the immune system problem? Scientists aren't yet sure, and it might depend on which immune system disorder we're talking about. But researchers are pretty sure there's a link. In general, if you have immune system problems, you are more likely to develop type 2 diabetes.

Do you have any known immune system problems?
❑ Yes   ❑ No

If you answer "yes," then be sure to talk with your doctor to find out more about how these problems may contribute to your diagnosis of prediabetes. Learn whether these conditions are apt to make type 2 diabetes more likely.

Speed Bump #3: Side Effects from Medications

Type 2 diabetes and certain medications are linked in a few ways:

- Some meds affect how your body processes or uses glucose.
- Some meds affect how your body makes or uses insulin.

The end results can be blood glucose levels that are too high. This chart summarizes some types of medications that can raise glucose levels and put you at risk.

SUBSTANCES THAT CAN RAISE BLOOD GLUCOSE LEVELS

Do you use any of the medications in the chart below?

❑ Yes   ❑ No   ❑ I don't know

If you answer "yes," speak with your doctor to find out more. These substances may be a factor in your prediabetes diagnosis—and may be putting you at greater risk for developing type 2 diabetes.

Medication	Why It's Used
Corticosteroids (used to treat inflammation)	To reduce inflammation, calm the immune system
Thiazides (diuretics or water pills)	To rid body of excess fluid, lowering blood pressure
Sympathomimetic agents (dobutamine or terbutaline)	To help the heart beat more effectively, or to prevent contractions during pregnancy
Antipsychotics	To treat mental health problems such as schizophrenia

Questions for Consideration

We've already gone through a list of questions above. For each "yes" answer, be sure to learn as much as you can about the risk and how it might be contributing to prediabetes. Ask your doctor what you can do—if anything—to counteract these risks. And don't forget to take a close look at Part III, where we'll have a chance to talk about how you can find routes to follow to minimize or eliminate these risks to your health.

5

DANGEROUS CURVES— LIFESTYLE RISKS

There's a curve exiting California Highway 1 on the way to Santa Cruz that natives fondly refer to as the "fish hook." It looks benign enough. But as you leave the freeway and make your way around it, the curve suddenly tightens. The barrier alongside the curve has dings and black marks from vehicles that have bashed into it by going too fast or too carelessly. These kinds of curves are relatively frequent in hilly country. But they still often surprise me. Luckily, so far I've watched my speed and managed to stay on the road...mostly. These tight curves are a little like lifestyle risks. It's how you take these curves from day to day that makes the difference between crashing and getting to your destination safe and sound.

Lifestyle factors include how you live day to day: What you eat. How much you eat. What you weigh. How active you are. And whether you're under a lot of stress. Let's take a closer look at these lifestyle factors and find out if they may play a role in *your* health.

The Most Dangerous Curve:
Your Weight and Why It Matters

You're cruising down the highway, making good time and enjoying the view, when suddenly you see a sign:

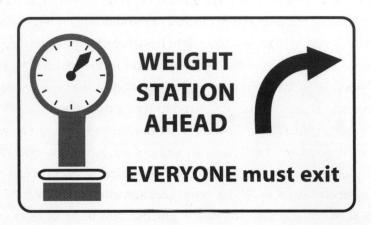

What the...? You dutifully pull off, roll through the in-motion scale, and stop to chat with the booth worker. Her smile turns to a frown as the weight of your vehicle registers. She shakes her head sadly at you and comments, "A bit too much. Better lose some of that load." And she directs you off to the left, onto the exit marked "Diabetesville Ahead."

Your own weight is determined by a combination of things:

- What, when, and how much you eat
- How your body uses the food that you eat
- Your level of physical activity

But what's the big deal about weight and its connection to prediabetes and diabetes? The concept is quite simple: Developing type 2 diabetes is most often associated with being overweight. But what is "overweight"? Just a couple of extra pounds? Obesity? Somewhere in between? And what about that recent news that people who weigh a little bit more don't drop dead as early as thin folks do?

It all comes down to a matter of location. That is, the location of your extra weight, which matters almost as much as the amount of weight you carry around on your frame. Researchers have noted that extra fat in the area of the abdomen is what seems to be linked to diabetes. You might have heard it called having an apple-shaped body—that is, being round in the middle. A pear-shaped body, where extra weight is carried in the hips and legs, seems to be less frequently linked to type 2 diabetes.

Let's take a closer look at the extra weight you might be lugging around. It's made up primarily of fat. And each pound of fat on your body is made up of 3,500 calories. So you can see how it adds up fast. The process goes something like this: When your blood contains too much glucose, the body does everything it can to get rid of it. Some of the glucose is put out as waste through the urine. A lot of it is changed into fat, the body's system of fuel storage, for later use. Over time, as more fat is stored and your weight rises, hormone levels shift. Your body makes more fat-producing and fat-storing hormones and fewer glucose-using hormones. The whole fat situation slowly spirals out of control, leaving you with extra pounds and associated problems such as diabetes.

Let's get even more specific and talk about *your* weight. First off, how much do you weigh? Is it too much? You can use the following Body Mass Index Chart to get a rough idea.

Step 1: Find your height on the left side of the chart.

Step 2: Follow along to the right until you find your weight.

Step 3: Go straight down from your weight to find your BMI in the bottom row.

Body Mass Index Chart

Height	Weight											
4'10"	96	100	105	110	115	119	124	129	134	138	143	
4'11"	94	99	104	109	114	119	124	128	133	138	143	148
5'0"	97	102	107	112	118	123	128	133	138	143	148	153
5'1"	100	106	111	116	122	127	132	137	143	148	153	158
5'2"	104	109	115	120	126	131	136	142	147	153	158	164
5'3"	107	113	118	124	130	135	141	146	152	158	163	169
5'4"	110	116	122	128	134	140	145	151	157	163	169	174
5'5"	114	120	126	132	138	144	160	156	162	168	174	180
5'6"	118	124	130	136	142	148	155	161	167	173	179	186
5'7"	121	127	134	140	146	153	159	166	172	178	185	191
5'8"	125	131	138	144	151	158	164	171	177	184	190	197
5'9"	128	135	142	149	155	162	169	176	182	189	196	203
5'10"	132	139	146	153	160	167	174	181	188	195	202	207
5'11"	136	143	150	157	165	172	179	186	193	200	208	215
6'0"	140	147	154	162	169	177	184	191	199	206	213	221
6'1"	144	151	159	166	174	182	189	197	204	212	219	227
6'2"	148	155	163	171	179	186	194	202	210	218	225	233
6'3"	152	160	168	176	184	192	200	208	216	224	232	240
6'4"	165	163	172	180	189	197	205	213	221	230	238	246
BMI	19	20	21	22	23	24	25	26	27	28	29	30

Step 1: Find your height on the left side of the chart.

Step 2: Follow along to the right until you find your weight.

Step 3: Go straight down from your weight to find your BMI on the bottom line.

WHAT IS YOUR BMI NUMBER? HERE'S WHAT IT MEANS:

If your BMI is . . .	. . . then you are
Less than 20	Underweight
20–24	At a desirable weight
25–29	Overweight
Greater than 29	Obese

Take me, for instance. I'm 5'4" and weigh 140 pounds on a good day. That puts my BMI at 24, the upper limit for desirable. My ideal weight range would be between 116 and 140. So if I put on any more weight (or weigh myself on a "bad" day), I'm heading for trouble.

Now about that apple–pear thing. Researchers have discovered an easy and surprisingly accurate way to assess your risk based on whether excess weight is around your middle (the apple image) or somewhere else (such as the pear). All you need is a long belt and two magic numbers:

35 for women and 40 for men

That's inches. You might even want to mark those lengths on the backside of the belt. Then simply measure yourself around the waist. Remember, we're talking about your *actual* waistline—around the belly button, not *under* or *over* that roll of you-know-what! Are you past the magic number? If so, your risk of developing diabetes increases. So does your risk of developing other health problems such as high blood pressure or heart disease.

Is your BMI 25 or higher?

❑ Yes   ❑ No   ❑ Can't figure it out

Is your waistline greater than 35 inches if you're a woman or 40 inches if you're a man?

❑ Yes   ❑ No

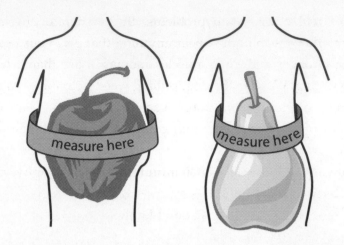

If you answer "yes" to either question, you *are* at great risk of developing diabetes, not to mention you're already at risk for cardiovascular problems. If you answer "no" to both questions, way to go! You have the most important risk factor for type 2 diabetes under control. Keep up the good work. If you can't figure out your BMI or don't quite trust the belt trick, ask your doctor to help.

The Next Dangerous Curve: Standing Still

You can probably guess one way that inactivity can be a risk factor for diabetes: Lack of physical activity can lead to weight gain, and you know from what you just read that having too much weight is a *big* risk factor. Also, inactivity may contribute to both insulin resistance and high levels of blood glucose. Remember, insulin resistance is the inability of insulin to lead glucose into the cells.

But what constitutes "inactivity"? Let's work backward from the general recommendation for healthy levels of activity. Most health care and diabetes experts suggest that you get at least 30 minutes of moderate physical activity on most days of the week. Anything less than that puts you at greater risk for diabetes and other health problems. By "moderate physical activity," they mean darned near anything that gets your heart beating stronger and your muscles moving more than when you're resting. Walking the dog, pulling weeds, climbing stairs, carrying groceries into the house, vacuuming the floor—all are examples of activities that could count toward the 30-minute total. So ask yourself:

Do you get LESS THAN 30 minutes of moderate physical activity on most days?

❑ Yes ❑ No ❑ I don't know

If you answer "yes," then you're at increased risk of developing diabetes. First off, your lack of activity makes it easier to gain weight. Second, your lack of activity may make insulin work less effectively in your body. If you answer "no," then congratulations! You're controlling one important risk factor. If you answer "I don't know," then find out. Track your activity for a couple of days. How much time are you at rest? How much are you on the move?

The Blind Curve: Stress

We could probably all add this risk factor to our "yes" list. After all, it takes a lot of emotional energy to deal with the daily events of life: job, family, finances, other health issues, and just plain growing older. Throw in a couple of extra, unexpected events, and *voilà!* You've got big-time stress. So what's the problem? Stress is a normal part of life, isn't it?

There is a connection between stress and diabetes. Some of it is direct, some less so. Here's how the two are linked:

- If you're always rushing around trying to meet all your commitments, you'll have little energy left for focusing on your health.

- Feeling stress for long periods can make your blood glucose levels go up.
- If you're feeling overwhelmed, it's less likely that you'll be able to take charge of managing your health.

So ask yourself this question:

Do you have often have high levels of stress in your life?
❑ Yes   ❑ No

If you answer "yes," then stress may be playing a role both in your diagnosis of prediabetes and in your risk for developing diabetes. If you answer "no," then you're one lucky person—or one healthy person. Keep on keeping the stress under control to prevent it from becoming another health risk for you.

Questions for Consideration

We've already asked the questions. Now take a look at all your answers. How are lifestyle issues impacting your health? Did you answer "yes" to any of the risks: being overweight, not getting enough physical activity, or feeling a lot of stress? All "yes" answers indicate a need for you to pay close attention to your life, so that you can find ways to prevent the things you do in your daily life from sending you dangerously around the bend closer to diabetes.

6

UNFORESEEN MECHANICAL BREAKDOWNS— "JUST BECAUSE" RISKS

Even if you keep your vehicle in good repair, sometimes bad stuff happens while you're driving down the road. You blow a tire. The radiator overheats. A water pump seizes up. Another car bumps into you. It's frustrating, because it's unanticipated and it delays your journey. But there wasn't much you could do to prevent these emergencies. You just have to gut it out and get the vehicle off the road and repaired. These "just because" risk factors are somewhat like that. You don't have much of a choice over your age, your ethnicity, or other "just because" factors. Nonetheless, these factors increase your risk of having prediabetes or developing type 2 diabetes. Why? Don't ask! Researchers have seen connections between these factors and developing diabetes. They don't necessarily know why the connection is there. Frustrating, to be sure. But, unfortunately, that's the way it is. Let's take a look at some of these factors.

Your Model Year

If you're a classic model—over age 60—then, like it or not, your risk for diabetes rises. Why? Perhaps the body has been dealing too long with processing high levels of glucose. Maybe your pancreas is simply starting to tire out. Your body might be needing fewer nutrients as it's slowing down, but you haven't adjusted your food intake to match. These are only possibilities. The reality is that there's a direct connection that needs to be taken seriously. So ask yourself:

Are you over age 60?

❏ Yes   ❏ No   ❏ I don't know (just kidding!)

If you answer "yes," then be sure to watch your other risks as well, especially since you've already been diagnosed with prediabetes. It could be a short trip to Diabetes Town if you're not careful. If you answer "no," then you're off the hook on this risk for now. But remember that your age will eventually catch up to you. If you have prediabetes now, take steps to manage it so that you won't have to worry about it so much when you hit the big six-oh.

Family Trouble

Diabetes does run in families, it seems. This may be because of inherited factors, or common lifestyle practices, or a combination of both. Scientists have gone to great lengths to try to tease out all the answers to this question, with varying success. What *is* known is that if a close blood relative such as a mother or father, grandparent, or sibling has diabetes, your risk is greater. So ask yourself these simple questions:

Did your mother have diabetes?

❏ Yes   ❏ No   ❏ I don't know

Do you have other close relatives who have diabetes?
❑ Yes   ❑ No   ❑ I don't know

If you answer "yes," to either question, then find out what you can about what led to their diabetes and what has helped them manage it. Your risk for developing diabetes is great—especially if your mother had the disease. If you answer "no," be glad that you have one less risk to worry about. If you "don't know," then find out! Ask your parents, grandparents, aunts, and uncles whether anyone in the family had or has diabetes. Remember that they may refer to it as "high sugar" or by another name.

Your Brand, Model, or Style

"Don't buy that kind of minivan," car-guy Dave told me recently. "They're having all kinds of transmission problems." Over a long period of time, certain models or brands of vehicles develop reputations for having specific problems. Unfortunately, the same is true for certain groups of people when it comes to their developing prediabetes or diabetes. Why? If you discover the link, pass the info on to your local diabetes professionals. They'll be pleased that someone finally figured it out! In the meantime, it's likely that certain ethnic, racial, or cultural groups are at greater risk because of a range of factors that all come together. They could include these:

- An inherited tendency toward diabetes
- Differences in how bodies create and use insulin and glucose
- Differences in immune system function
- Adopting new foods and practices when coming to a new country
- Leaving behind foods and practices from the "old country"
- Unavailability of healthier food choices

A lot of other factors could also be involved. In the United States, groups that have a higher than "average" rate of diabetes include the following:

- African Americans
- Hispanic/Latino Americans
- Asian/Pacific Islander Americans
- Native Americans

Do you belong to a group of people that have a higher risk of developing diabetes?
❑ Yes   ❑ No

If you answer "yes," you might be tempted to feel discouraged. After all, you have no control over which ethnic group you belong to. But remember, it's not guaranteed that you will develop diabetes. The point is to be aware of the increased risk so that you can take steps to deal with it and stay on the road to good health. If you answer "no," then you can be glad that you have one less risk for developing diabetes. But don't get cocky! If you already have prediabetes, you'll need to do all you can to understand and deal with your other risks.

Prior Run-ins with Diabetes: Gestational Diabetes

I just got a letter from my friend Kathy, updating me on her life back in my hometown. Kathy told me that her daughter, who had diabetes while pregnant with her one child over 15 years ago, has recently been diagnosed with type 2. I was distressed to hear the news, but not particularly surprised. Luckily, her daughter generally leads a healthy lifestyle and is taking her diagnosis seriously.

You, too, probably know women who acquired diabetes while pregnant. Perhaps you did, as well. This type of diabetes is referred to as gestational diabetes.

Why does it happen? The causes aren't well understood. During pregnancy, incredible changes occur in the immune system and the hormone system, both of which are also involved in the development of diabetes. Weight gain is also common—and expected—during pregnancy, posing another risk factor for diabetes.

It is known that certain groups of women are at greater risk of developing gestational diabetes (also called GDM, or gestational diabetes mellitus). These include:

- African Americans
- Hispanic/Latino Americans
- Native Americans
- Women who are overweight
- Women with a family history of diabetes
- Women who have a pregnancy later in life

It's bad enough to have to deal with the potential problems associated with gestational diabetes, including miscarriage, birth defects, death of the fetus, and the increased likelihood that the child will eventually develop diabetes or obesity as well. Women with gestational diabetes are also more likely to develop high blood pressure during pregnancy. They're more likely to end up needing a C-section. And—following the theme of this part of the book—women who have had gestational diabetes are much more at risk of developing diabetes within five to ten years, even if the diabetes went away after birth. That's in addition to the 10 percent of women with gestational diabetes who remain diabetic after the birth of their child.

Have you ever had diabetes while pregnant?
❑ Yes   ❑ No   ❑ I don't know

If you answer "yes," you are definitely at increased risk for developing diabetes. Take this risk seriously! If you answer "no," then be thankful you have one less risk to worry about. And if you "don't know," try to check back into your medical records to find out. If your baby was more than nine pounds at birth, you may have had diabetes. If you did have gestational diabetes, your chances of acquiring type 2 diabetes are greater. The time to take action is now, before you reach that diagnosis.

 About 7 percent of pregnancies in the U.S. are accompanied by gestational diabetes. It's a fact that women with gestational diabetes experience a higher rate of fetal death and stillbirth. There's some evidence that the same problems occur at a higher rate in *women with prediabetes* as well.

Questions for Consideration

You've already answered a number of questions above about your "just because" factors—areas you often had nothing to do with and can rarely change. But even though you can't control your age, ethnic background, past medical history, and such, it's important for you to be aware of these factors. They're often huge influencers on how you deal with managing prediabetes and delaying or even preventing diabetes. For instance, your ethnic background may influence your attitude about weight or the kinds of foods you eat. We'll talk a lot more about all this in Part III.

7

THE DIABETES– CARDIOVASCULAR CUTOFF: SYNDROME X

I love taking those cutoffs from the highway to out-of-the-way towns, even if it takes me longer to reach my destination. On some of my favorite cutoffs, such as a back route into the Lake Tahoe area, we've noticed historical mile markers along the way. Unfortunately, there's one cutoff on Prediabetes Way that you'd really rather avoid. And that's <u>Syndrome X</u>. What is it? Do you have it?

Syndrome X is the name originally given to a group of risk factors that researchers discovered puts a person at greater risk of developing several serious health problems. Recently, researchers have tried to rename this syndrome to better reflect what it means. <u>Metabolic Syndrome</u> and <u>Insulin Resistance Syndrome</u> are the two phrases most in fashion at the moment. Whatever you call it, persons with Syndrome X risk factors seem to be at greater risk of developing diabetes, cardiovascular problems such as heart attacks and strokes, and other chronic health problems (such as kidney or eye problems) that are associated with these two diseases.

Assessing many of these risk factors requires blood tests. If you don't have a family doctor or health insurance, you can still find ways to have these tests done at little or no cost. Health fairs and drugstores offer many of these tests for low fees, or for free. Your county's health department may also be able to recommend ways to have these tests done that won't break your budget.

We've actually talked about all the factors involved in Syndrome X/Metabolic Syndrome in the preceding chapters. So why bring it up here? Is Syndrome X a real problem, or just a dramatic way to get your attention? Maybe both. Listen to this: More than 40 million folks in the United States may have Metabolic Syndrome. Are you one of them? Frankly, if you've been diagnosed with prediabetes, you're likely to qualify for the Metabolic Syndrome label as well. But just to be sure, take a look at these mile markers along the way, to see if these risks apply to you.

Mile Marker 1: Are you "obese"?

Remember that belt trick from Chapter 5? For women, this means your waistline is greater than 35 inches. For men, it means your waistline is greater than 40 inches. You can also use the body mass index (BMI) to determine obesity. Skip back to Chapter 5 for more details.

Mile Marker 2: Do you have glucose intolerance or insulin resistance?

Check those blood glucose numbers from Chapter 4. If your blood glucose levels from either the fasting glucose test or the glucose challenge test are within the "impaired" range, then you're glucose intolerant (your body can't use all the glucose in your bloodstream) or insulin resistant (your body's insulin isn't working to get the glucose into your cells).

Mile Marker 3: Do you have high blood pressure, high LDL (bad) cholesterol, and high levels of triglycerides (a type of fat found in blood)?

Okay, we need a little more explanation here. We've talked earlier about cardiovascular problems arising from diabetes. Cardiovascular health is measured in many ways, including by tracking your blood pressure and levels of different types of fats in your blood.

Let's start with blood pressure. This is the force created in your blood vessels from the blood flowing through them. Blood pressure is measured two ways:

- While the heart is beating (systolic)
- While the heart is between beats (diastolic)

You'll see this written as two numbers, the systolic on top and the diastolic on the bottom:

$$\frac{130 \text{ mm Hg}}{80 \text{ mm Hg}}$$
      Systolic Blood Pressure
      Diastolic Blood Pressure

The abbreviation "mm Hg" stands for "millimeters of mercury." This measurement comes from the "old days" when blood pressure was measured by how high your pressure pushed mercury up a tube.

What about *your* blood pressure? Do you know what it is? Ask your doctor to tell you, the next time you have it taken. Or go to any number of places—health fairs, drugstores, a friend who has her own high blood pressure measuring kit—to get it measured for free. Use this chart to find the ranges. There's also space to record your own blood pressure.

If your own blood pressure is 130/80 or higher (that is, within the "prehypertensive" category or higher), you're considered at risk for Metabolic Syndrome.

Blood Pressure Levels			
Level	Systolic	Diastolic	What It Means
Low	Less than 120 mm Hg	Less than 80 mm Hg	You have a reduced risk of heart disease and kidney disease
Prehyper-tensive	120–139 mm Hg	80–89 mm Hg	If you already have prediabetes, you're at increased risk of heart attack, stroke, and other problems associated with blood vessel damage
Hypertensive	140 mm Hg or higher	90 mm Hg or higher	You're at increased risk of heart attack, stroke, artery disease, eye problems, kidney problems, and nerve problems
At risk for Metabolic Syndrome	130 mg Hg or greater	80 mm Hg or greater	
Your blood pressure			

Now for LDL cholesterol. The technical name is low-density lipoprotein. You've probably heard it called "bad" cholesterol. Think of LDL as a special wrapper around chunks of fat to help the fat flow through your blood vessels. The problem is, LDLs often clump up and get stuck in blood vessels, especially in blood vessels already damaged by high blood pressure or high levels of blood glucose. This makes it harder for blood to circulate easily through your body and causes even more damage and even higher blood pressure.

Here's a chart to show the various levels of LDL cholesterol. There's also space to record your own LDL level. If you don't know your LDL cholesterol level, ask your doctor for past results, or get it checked as soon as possible!

LDL Cholesterol Levels		
Normal	At Risk	Your Number
Less than 100 mg/dL	Greater than 100 mg/dL	

You might notice that the numbers here are either "normal" or "at risk." In other publications, you may see the terms "borderline high," "high," and "very high" also used. That's because those ranges were developed for people who didn't have to worry about prediabetes or diabetes. But when you add higher than normal blood glucose levels to the picture, your risk jumps up more quickly.

Finally, there are triglycerides, a type of fat found in your blood. Triglycerides come from the food you eat. In addition, your body can make triglycerides from other substances. High levels of triglycerides can block your arteries. It's also known that people with diabetes and prediabetes tend to have higher levels of triglycerides than the rest of us folks. Ask your doctor for your most recent triglycerides results, or have the test done soon. It's often done together with standard cholesterol tests. Here's a breakdown of the range of triglyceride results.

Triglyceride Levels		
Normal	At Risk	Your Number
Less than 150 mg/dL	Greater than 150 mg/dL	

As with LDL cholesterol, because you have prediabetes, as soon as you rise above the "normal" category you're at greater risk of cardiovascular problems and Metabolic Syndrome.

So let's summarize "Mile Marker 3." If your numbers for blood pressure, LDL cholesterol, and triglycerides are ALL greater than normal, you're at greater risk for the health conditions associated with Metabolic Syndrome.

Mile Marker 4: Do you have low HDL (good) cholesterol?

HDL cholesterol is otherwise known as high-density lipoprotein or "good" cholesterol. Like LDL, HDL is another "wrapper" to help fat move through the blood vessels. Unlike LDL, you *want* high levels of HDL in your blood. That's because HDL pulls junk out of the bloodstream, including clumped-up LDLs. So you're in trouble if you have too few HDLs to do the clean-up job. Here's a chart for HDL. If you don't know your HDL level, ask your doctor for past results, or get it checked soon.

HDL Cholesterol Levels		
Normal	At Risk	Your Number
Greater than 40 mg/dL	Less than 40 mg/dL	

If your HDL level falls into the "at risk" category, then you're at greater risk of developing the health conditions associated with Metabolic Syndrome.

Questions for Consideration

If you answer "yes" to ALL these mile markers, then you're a member of the Syndrome X Club or, if you prefer, the Metabolic Syndrome Society. That means you're at greater risk of developing diabetes, cardiovascular problems, and other chronic health conditions. But don't despair! Just look at it as extra motivation to drive your health in a new direction. If you didn't answer "yes" to all these questions, then take a moment to congratulate yourself on keeping some very important risk factors under control. But remember that because you already have prediabetes, your risk for these problems is greater than it would be for the average healthy Joe or Jane.

If you qualify for Metabolic Syndrome status, what should you do? With all the media hype about Syndrome X and such, you'd think that there must be a detailed medical plan to deal with this condition. Actually, the solution is simply stated: Lose weight. Of course, doing it is tougher. So that's why you'll want to read on. Many of the routes you can take to manage prediabetes in Part III are the same things you'll need to do to avoid the Metabolic Syndrome cutoff to diabetes and cardiovascular problems.

PART III

*Your Travel Plan
for Good Health*

So far you've learned about the slow, winding, bumpy road from health, to prediabetes, to type 2 diabetes. You've identified some of the risks that may have led you to prediabetes and that could lead you on to the very jarring Diabetes Street and other serious health problems. And you've discovered reasons to turn back toward a healthier route.

What's next for you?

Your primary destination is to find ways to help your body work more effectively to get glucose from your blood into your cells. But, like any good road trip, it helps to develop a travel plan before you make your next move. This part of the book will serve as that plan. You can move down many potential routes, yet trying them all at once can become overwhelming. Where to start? Ultimately, that's for you to decide. This travel plan includes information about:

- Developing a **healthy attitude** (Chapter 8)
- **Setting goals** and selecting approaches for managing your weight (Chapter 9)
- **Eating your way** to good health (Chapter 10)

- Fitting **physical activity** into your plan (Chapter 11)
- How **medication**—including diabetes medications, other medications, and even supplements—might help (Chapter 12)
- **Other steps you can take**, including getting regular health exams, setting up your own prediabetes support team, monitoring glucose levels at home, taking steps toward heart health, watching out for complications, and overcoming barriers to change (Chapter 13)

My guess is that most folks will gain the greatest benefit by taking a straight-on-through route, starting with Chapter 9 through Chapter 11. In Chapters 12 and 13 you'll find bits and pieces of strategies you can put together as needed to help you along your way.

8

DEVELOP A HEALTHY ATTITUDE

Dealing with a little stress along your daily journey through life? Feeling overwhelmed? Maybe even feeling a little depressed or hopeless, wondering if there's really anything you can do to get yourself back on the right road to health? Or perhaps worrying that you simply have a bad attitude—thinking that you have neither time nor patience for dealing with this so-called health condition called prediabetes? You can begin to deal with these questions by acknowledging one fact right from the start:

Stress happens.

And, like the more famous saying (you know—the one with the four-letter word) about things that happen, sometimes all these stressful feelings and related stuff keep piling higher and higher.

Unfortunately, feeling all this yucky stuff isn't going to help you shift gears from prediabetes back toward health. Instead, your attitude toward the stressful stuff in your life can nudge you closer toward type 2 diabetes in ways like these:

- **Feeling rushed** to meet all your commitments leaves little energy for yourself and your needs, and can end up with your feeling overwhelmed.

- **Feeling overwhelmed** by too many tasks and responsibilities makes it less likely that you'll take charge of your health, and leaves you feeling stressed.
- **Feeling stressed** for long periods can make your blood glucose levels rise *and* can lead to depression.
- **Feeling depressed** can keep you from taking any action to improve your health or your life.

You can detour around all these potential potholes by taking some time now to develop a healthy state of mind. That's why this chapter comes first in the travel plan. If you develop a healthy attitude toward both your life and your prediabetes, then making other changes won't seem quite so overwhelming or even impossible. Let's take a look at some of those stops along Attitude Way.

Stop 1: Identify the Stressors in Your Life

I live off an old farm road in earthquake country. So bumps and cracks and small slippages in the road seem normal to me. I wouldn't know what to do if the pavement was smooth, if I didn't pop a tire every so often on the edge of a pothole, or have to drive around a pile of dirt that just slid down the hillside. Stressors are like those little troubles in the road, the individual things that make life just a bit more trying. Each small hole or slide or crack is annoying, but perhaps not such a big deal. If you're traveling over bumpy pavement all the time, however, you end up feeling shaken, tired, and frustrated. Added together, these "little" stressors can make life downright unpleasant. Worst case, the stressors can become depressors, leading you to simply give up. We don't want to go there, so let's start by figuring out just what potholes lie in wait in *your* road of life. Use this checklist as a guide. There's plenty of space to add any more that you may discover.

Your Personal Potholes	
Stressors	**How They Can Affect You**
Prediabetes diagnosis	• Feeling overwhelmed by the thought of developing diabetes • Feeling like you've lost control of your health and your life • Worries about the future • Wondering whether it's true and whether it will progress toward diabetes • Frustrated about where to start to get back to health
Other health conditions	• Feeling like you've lost control of your health and your life • Worries about the future • Wondering whether your prediabetes or other diagnoses are true • Frustrated about where to start to get back to health
Your job	• Concern about doing your job well • Feeling stress about deadlines • Worries about whether prediabetes will prevent you from performing your job well • Worries that you might lose your job if you go on to develop diabetes • Worries that your employer might not consider the difference between a diagnosis of prediabetes and a diagnosis of diabetes
Family responsibilities	• Concern over being able to fulfill your responsibilities as a member of your family • Frustration over lack of understanding or support from other family members • Anxiety about making the entire family follow changes that would help you regain your health
Finances	• Concern about how you might pay for costs associated with prediabetes • Concern about how the economy of your area will affect your ability to earn an income
Other life changes— good and bad	• Feeling overwhelmed • Having thoughts preoccupied with the changes • Wondering how the changes will affect your health

Stop 2: Gear Up to Improve Your Attitude

You're driving down the road, you hit a hole, and the car veers off the pavement. What do you do? End up backward in the middle of a lettuce patch, like I did once? I hope not! Now that you know what your personal potholes are, you can select responses that can reduce their impact on your life *and* your health. You'll need a two-gear response:

1. Take immediate evasive action.
2. Check your compass.

For your car, you'd take immediate action to stop it from going off the road. Then you'd want to be sure to get your bearings so you can avoid similar problems in the future: Remember where that hole is, for example. Then you can call the road crew to fix it, steer slightly around it, slow down, or even take a driving course to better learn how to avoid these holes. Personal potholes need to be dealt with in the same way. You need to respond with both gears to stop the stressor from messing up your life and your health. How? Let's start with immediate action.

Stop 3: Take Immediate Action

Keep a toolkit of stress-relieving techniques close at hand so that you can use them whenever you notice the tension level rising. Right when you recognize the feelings that the stressor creates in you, stop immediately and try one of these techniques:

Breathe it away. Close your eyes. Through your nose, take a long, slow, deep breath, letting the air fill your chest. Hold it for a few seconds. Slowly let the air out through your mouth. Repeat this a couple of times.

Take a laugh pill. The saying "laughter is the best medicine" is backed by sound scientific evidence. Laughing relieves stress—and improves your health. Have quick access to something that makes you laugh, or at least smile. Perhaps a book of jokes, a funny calendar, a cute photo of your grandkids or pets. Make sure you get at least one good laugh in before returning to your activities.

Shrug it off. A quick stretch can help you shrug off stress, especially if it tends to build up in your body. Raise your shoulders up toward your ears. Hold this position for a few seconds. Then lower them. Repeat several times.

Nod off. Yes, a catnap would be nice, but that's not what I mean. Instead, relieve body tension in your neck by gently leaning your head to the left, nodding down to the center and rolling up to the right. Then nod back down to the center and up to the left. Bring your head back to center, and you're ready for the next round of activity.

Make a quick getaway. It's okay to zone out for a few minutes! Keep a novel handy—or even a movie if you're near a video or DVD player. When things are getting too tense, step out, sit down, and read a few pages or view your show for a few minutes.

Listen up. Music can help you deal with the hustle and bustle around you. Sometimes you need music to rev you up. But mostly, you could probably use some tunes that soothe your soul. A lullaby may not be appropriate when there's work to be done, but you can find music that fits in with your setting that will also ease the stress of your day. Experiment to find out what works best for you: Borrow music CDs or tapes from friends. Or check them out from the library. Consider styles you might not normally choose. Classical, easy listening, new age, jazz, folk, and most other styles of music all have selections that can help you keep your cool.

Take a mental trip. Choose your favorite restful place—the mountains, by a stream, at the beach, wherever. Close your eyes and picture yourself there. Involve all your senses: What do you see? Feel? Smell? Hear? After a few minutes, come back to the "real world" refreshed.

Get wet. It's amazing how a warm bath or a quick steaming shower can wash away more than just the dirt. Stressful feelings can go down the drain, too. Add a little lavender or other relaxing bath scent, or use a fragrant body wash.

Play with your kids. Or grandkids. Or the neighbor's kids. Or, in a pinch, a pet. Concentrate all your efforts on playing like they do. Follow their lead. Whether it's tag, baseball, Barbies, GameBoy, or fetch, if you do it with them *their* way, you're bound to leave yourself (and your stress) behind. And you might just find that your playmates calm down, too, as they come to appreciate your undivided attention.

Savor sighs and yawns. These are your body's natural attempts to relax. Think about it: When you sigh or yawn, you breathe in deeply, breathe out slowly and fully, and pause for just a few moments before beginning your "regular" breathing pattern again. So next time you feel a yawn coming on, take it as a sign that you need to relax. Don't stifle it! Go with the yawn. And let yourself sigh when you need to. Try two or three sighs in a row, even. Notice how much more relaxed you feel immediately afterward.

You probably have more stress relievers to add. Just remember: Do it! Right away.

Stop 4: Consult Your Compass

Quick stress relievers are great for the moment. They keep you on the road and avoid a crash. But you also need some long-term strategies, like a compass to keep yourself grounded and sane as you're navigating the responsibilities, activities, and concerns in your life, including prediabetes. Your health care team, employer-sponsored workshops, and community organizations may all provide help with these and other strategies.

Determine your top values. What's this got to do with avoiding stress? Several years ago, I was definitely feeling stressed out: I had recently divorced, was trying to decide whether to move closer to family in another state, and didn't know what to do about my career. So I sat down and listed the values that were most important to me in my life. Those values guided me through the next year or so. But then I got caught up in events that seemed to happen without my control, and even-

Gaining Support for Depression

 Everyone feels stress and frustration now and then. But when blue turns into black, your family and friends may not be able to help enough. You might need some serious support from health care professionals. You could be suffering from depression if you're feeling any of the following:

- You can't make decisions.
- You feel hopeless.
- You're always sleepy, yet have trouble sleeping.

Depression may be initiated by the stressful events in your life. But it's actually a medical problem—an imbalance of brain chemicals. It may not go away unless you get professional medical help. A combination of medication and therapy usually does the trick. If you think you may be depressed, see your primary care doctor right away. Get a referral for help, so that you can once again travel with pleasure, even when you're dealing with such serious concerns as prediabetes.

tually found myself feeling depressed, drained, not knowing what to do. One day, just for fun, I dug through a pile of notes I'd written over the years. Guess what I found? That earlier list of values. I realized that even though my circumstances had changed a lot, my values had not. It was time once again to make choices in my life based on what I valued the most. Want to know what they were? Spending lots of time with family and friends, helping others however I can, having a home of my own, and being creative in as many ways as I can. Not necessarily revolutionary, but important to me. Your values are likely to be different. The point is, figure out what they are—and don't forget to honor them! I don't think I will anymore. Sticking to those values makes it easier to find your way through just about anything, allowing both you and your health to thrive.

Assess your priorities. Sometimes you have to admit that you just can't do it all. Something's got to give. And you have to accept that that's okay. A hard one, I know—something I personally struggle with a lot. How do you make those tough choices? When do you know that "enough's enough"? This is where priorities come in. Priorities are based on values, with a little reality thrown in, such as earning an income to pay the bills. They're also *yours,* not someone else's, although it probably seems like there are plenty of folks around who are more than willing to place their priorities on your list! That's why it's a good step to take a look at priorities from time to time:

1. List all the priorities in your life.
2. Describe why each is important to you.
3. Rank the entire list, from top (#1) to bottom.
4. Decide what you can do with each priority: drop it, keep it, or change it. "Drop it" doesn't mean you lose it forever. Perhaps someone else can take it on. Perhaps you can

return to it someday when you have more time and energy. "Keep it" means it's part of the core of your life. "Change it" means you want to maintain the priority, but maybe in a different form. Do less of it, or assign it a lower rank, for example.

5. If you're thinking about changing a priority, note *how* you think it could be changed.

Review your list from time to time, and make any other changes to reflect any new goals and values you've identified.

Talk about it. Talk is cheap, they say. But it's also one essential component of destressing your life. You need to talk. But how, and to whom? That depends on your own personal style, your comfort level, the people closest to you, and the resources available in your community. Here are some possibilities:

- **Find a support group.** Frankly, there aren't a lot of groups specifically for people dealing with prediabetes; still, you can benefit from any group that focuses on healthy lifestyles or even type 2 diabetes. Local chapters of the American Diabetes Association, local and regional diabetes centers, hospitals, and large health care providers often sponsor support groups. Such groups give you a chance to voice your concerns to others who have probably gone through similar experiences. They can also offer you suggestions, a willing ear, and friendship. Look for support groups led by a professional such as a diabetes nurse, a medical social worker, or a counselor. Or you may find groups led by community health workers, knowledgeable nonprofessionals within your community who serve as bridges between patients and the sometimes baffling health care system.

- **Choose one-on-one counseling.** A group can be reassuring, but often you can benefit more from working individually with a trained counselor who has professional credentials, such as MSW, MA, MS, PhD, MD, or other designation. It may take a few sessions to know if you have a good match. If not, don't feel bad about looking for another person. A counselor can help you pinpoint whether you're experiencing serious levels of depression and can recommend a psychiatrist (an MD trained in psychology and able to prescribe medication), if medication to treat depression might be appropriate.
- **Go online.** The American Diabetes Association, other diabetes and health organizations, and even online service providers such as AOL and Yahoo offer bulletin boards, discussion groups, and chats for people dealing with prediabetes or diabetes.
- **Bend an ear.** Got a few good friends? A loyal sister or brother? Take advantage of the people close to you. When you're frustrated, be sure you check in with them, even it it's just to vent for a minute or two.

Pick your pleasure. A great, long-term stress reliever is simply to involve yourself in activities you enjoy. Hobbies such as model train building, activities such as swimming or gardening, and pursuits such as travel or participating in a book club can all provide pleasure, keep you physically active, and—the bonus—relieve stress.

Get support for your prediabetes travel plan. Assess how the people in your life influence your stress levels, both positively and negatively. Then think about how you can work with them more effectively to create a more peaceful attitude and environment around you. Make a list of the important people in your life. Then note how each of them helps you maintain your health—such as provides chances for laughter or trusts you on the job. Then list any ways in which they *don't* help you maintain your health, such as don't understand your need to make changes in your diet, or have a lot of their own problems to deal with. Then list what you can both do to make the relationship even better and more helpful to your health.

Questions for Consideration

Just like your car needs regular oil changes every couple of months, do yourself a favor and conduct a monthly "stress check." Take a minute or two to remember your values and priorities. Think about what you're feeling right now:

- What makes you happy?
- What makes you sad?
- What is frustrating you?
- What is worthwhile?

As long as you stay in touch with yourself, you'll be able to avoid those personal potholes—and when you do hit a stressor from time to time, you'll be better able to deal with it. Over time, lower levels of stress will ease the burden on your body, helping to lower those blood glucose levels and improve your overall health and well-being.

9

WATCH YOUR WEIGHT

"Heavier vehicles are safer," many folks maintain, as they hop into their armored tanks and chug off down the road. For me, the human equivalent is "Put a little more fat on those bones." I remember one of my aunts telling me often, "You're too skinny to be healthy!" Don't I wish I had that problem now... My aunt was wrong. I *didn't* need to put more fat on my bones. I'll bet you probably had an aunt—or a grandmother or mother or another relative—who told you the same thing.

If your weight falls within a desirable range (see Body Mass Index, page 52), then perhaps you can move on to another chapter. But if you've got prediabetes, it's highly likely that your weight is in the upper ranges ("overweight" or "obese") or at the high end of the "desirable" range, like me. And that extra weight can be hard on your system. You'll gain sizable benefits from any weight loss—even if it's only a few pounds. Working toward a desirable weight level eases your body's food-processing workload. Losing weight also helps "reteach" your body how to manage glucose levels in a way that doesn't damage your body or your health.

Bookstores and the airwaves are full of plans for losing weight. You may have tried a few—with little or no success, or with short-term loss that didn't last. Your destination this time is to make weight loss last for the long run. How? Don't even think about doing it all at once! That approach can be overwhelming and keep you from taking any steps at all. Besides, rapid weight loss is unhealthy—a shock to your system. Instead, look at weight loss as a three-part process:

1. **Stabilize your weight.** Stop the pounds from inching higher year after year.
2. Then begin to **lower your weight** to a healthier level.
3. Once you've reached an appropriate level, your goal is to **maintain that weight** for the long run.

Yes, you'll probably always have that third goal in the back of your mind. And that's okay. But if you focus on reaching the intermediate goals (steps 1 and 2), you'll be rewarded with steady progress that can keep you motivated for the long haul. Remember that old fable of the tortoise and the hare? The tortoise won by simply keeping on keeping on, and so will you if you mimic his approach.

How will you know when you've arrived at your weight-loss destination? Many health experts suggest that you aim for losing about 5 to 10 percent of your total body weight. For me, for example, that would be between 7 and 14 pounds. Let's go for the middle of that range: 7 percent. The first chart uses me for an example. The second chart is for you to fill out.

Now that you have a destination in mind, what do you need to do to arrive there? Plan to lose the weight over a period of at least 6 months—about 24 weeks. To find your weekly weight-loss destination, take the total number of pounds you want to lose and divide by 24. For me, that means losing just under half a pound per week. That's a goal I think I can achieve. Fill in the boxes on the next page to find your goal.

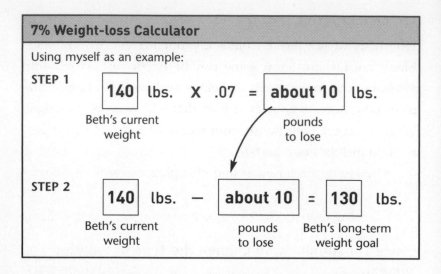

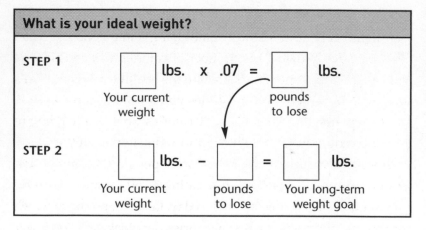

If the amount per week is more than one pound, then divide the total number of pounds by more weeks—36 or even 52 weeks, for example. This will give you a realistic goal.

Which Route to Choose?

Hundreds of weight-loss plans cry out for you to "try me!" Many are just fine, but some can be dangerous. Work with someone who understands diabetes—such as a dietitian or diabetes educator—to develop a plan that will work best for you. Whatever route you choose, your means of getting to your destination includes two parts:

- Lowering the number and changing the type of calories you eat.
- Getting more exercise.

Lower the Number and Change the Type of Calories You Eat

Diet. Don't you hate that word? I do. But whatever you call it, you'll probably need to make some changes in the food you eat. This includes reducing the number of calories you consume as well as selecting those foods that are the healthiest for you. Let's start with how many fewer calories you'll need to consume.

One pound of body fat is 3,500 calories. So if you're going to lose a pound a week, you'll need to reduce your diet by 3,500 calories per week. That's 500 calories per day. Losing a half pound a week would take your eating 1,750 calories less food per week—250 fewer calories each day. Losing 2 pounds a week would mean eating 7,000 fewer calories per week, or 1,000 fewer calories per day.

For most people, two main eating strategies can help you reach your weight-loss destination. The first one, reducing both saturated and trans fats in your diet, gets the biggest bang for the buck. That's because all fats create more fuel (and, thus, more calories) than equivalent amounts of protein or carbohydrate, as you'll see in the chart below. In particular, saturated fat (which comes mostly from animal sources) and trans fat (from the process of hydrogenation, making oils more solid) are bad news. Not only are they laden with calories, but they also wreck your heart and arteries. Along with reducing fat, you'll need to learn the second main eating strategy: how to choose your carbs wisely. Going for fresh (as in produce) and whole (as in grains) is a broad guideline to follow. How do you do this? Chapter 9 gives lots more specifics.

Gaining Support for Your Weight-Loss Plan

 You're probably tired of being harassed about your weight. You know your spouse, your mom, another relative, friends, even co-workers really do want to help—but all the nagging does is get you mad. What can you do about it? Whoever these naggers may be, acknowledge that they care about you and want to help. They just don't know how. You can help them turn their nagging into support you can use. Try some of these suggestions:

- Explain that you're trying to become healthier, but that it takes time to make changes.

- Describe the range of changes you need to make in order to get your blood glucose levels down to normal, then ask them to repeat in their own words.

- Point out specific actions they can take to help you. Examples: Offering to watch the kids so you can get out to walk. Not always insisting that you have second helpings. Learning more about healthy eating and food preparation—so that everyone can benefit. Joining with you as a weight-loss buddy.

- Offer "hard-core" naggers a choice: Either they respect your request for constructive support, or they keep their mouths shut. Don't forget to smile sweetly!

Calories of Food Components	
Component	Calories Per Gram
Fat	9
Protein	4
Carbohydrate	4

If you have concerns about not being able to lose weight through your diet, be sure to talk with your health care team. They can help you pinpoint roadblocks and suggest alternative routes. And remember that the next chapter offers ways in which you can use food to lower your weight while lowering your blood glucose levels.

Get More Exercise

Does exercise really help with weight loss? The answer is... (let's pause while I open the sealed envelope) YES. The difference may not seem dramatic, but exercise and changes in what you eat *together* often lead to successful weight loss. Exercise is even more helpful in keeping off the pounds once you've lost them. It makes sense that when your body's working hard, it burns up more calories, both during and immediately after exercise. Even more, think about where your body stores extra glucose: In your *muscles*. When those muscles move regularly, they use up the stored glucose and then signal to your body to send along more. Your body responds by pulling more glucose out of your blood vessels. Overall, glucose levels remain lower and more stable. But that's not all—the news about exercise gets even better: When you exercise regularly, levels of bad fats in your blood go down. Let's sum up the value of exercise like this: Regularly physical activity causes your metabolic and cardiovascular systems to operate more efficiently and effectively, placing less overall stress on your body. Exercise can also be a good stress reliever, and, as we talked about earlier, stress can make glucose levels soar higher.

Exercise offers other benefits that we'll talk about in Chapter 11. But for now you're wondering what kind and how much exercise you need. The short answer is this:

Probably more than you're getting now.

Okay, the "real" answer is this:

An accumulation of 30 minutes of moderate physical activity on most days.

So ask yourself: Am I physically active at least this amount every day? If you answer "yes," then you're using exercise as an effective tool to aid your weight control plan. If you answer "no," then it's time to make your move. Pay attention to Chapter 11 to find out more about what moderate physical activity is and how to add it into your daily routine along the road to better health.

Questions for Consideration

At each doctor's appointment, be sure to check in about your weight. You can also check your own progress at home, but don't get obsessed with it! Standing on the scales every morning can be downright demoralizing. Go for once a week, at most. Use the Weight-Loss Record below to track your progress.

You can also use that belt trick you might have tried in Chapters 5 and 7. All you need is that belt and the two magic numbers: 35 inches for women and 40 inches for men. The closer you get to that magic number, and to getting that belt around your thinner waist, the closer you are to your weight-loss goal.

If the idea of measuring your waistline turns you off, don't worry. Here are some other ways to monitor your progress. Ask yourself these questions:

Your Weight-Loss Record

Starting Weight	Starting BMI #	Long-term goal	Number of lbs. to lose

Date	Weight	Notes

- Have you stopped gaining weight?
- Are you losing weight, even if it's only a pound every week or so?
- Are your clothes getting "bigger" on you?
- Is your blood glucose level getting closer to normal?
- Is your blood pressure getting closer to normal?
- Do you feel better?
- Have you reached your weight-loss goal?
- If you've reached your goal, are you maintaining your weight?

Even one "yes" answer means that you *are* making progress toward weight loss. If you answer "yes" to more than one, be proud of your accomplishments and keep on working toward the ultimate goal: maintaining normal glucose levels and improved health. And don't forget to check the next two chapters for suggestions about using food and exercise to manage weight and control diabetes.

10

EATING YOUR WAY TO GOOD HEALTH

Seems like food can be your best friend—or your worst enemy—doesn't it? Can't live without it, can't live with too much of it, either. Talk about a narrow path to navigate! Most of us find the whole subject a bit frustrating. But what about my friend, Rich, who was gaining success as the owner of a specialty chocolate business when he got the diagnosis: *diabetes*. After falling into a bit of a funk for a while, he took the drastic step of shutting down his business and moving on to another career. Most of us with prediabetes don't have to feel forced into such dramatic steps—especially if we start now to do something about the food we eat.

The Link between Food and Prediabetes

We talked earlier about how the body converts the food you eat into glucose to fuel the cells. And you know that problems with this process can lead to prediabetes and, eventually, to diabetes. Eating too much can, over time, lead to the weight gain that is often linked to diabetes.

Making wise food choices can have positive benefits on your health, too. The food you eat can help you:

- Maintain adequate levels of nutrients for health and energy
- Stabilize or even lose weight
- Maintain blood glucose levels in a normal range
- Lower your risk of cardiovascular problems

What makes the difference between food helping your body and food being a troublemaker? Here are some of the factors involved:

- How many carbohydrates you eat
- What the carbs you eat are made up of (the combination of sugar, starch, and fiber)
- What kind of cooking or other processing has occurred
- What other food components have been eaten at the same time, such as fat, fiber, or other substances that speed or slow digestion
- What your blood glucose level was before you ate

You can manipulate these factors—through the food choices you make—to keep your blood glucose levels heading back down toward normal. That's your "big picture" goal. Sounds reasonably simple, doesn't it? The complication comes in realizing that everyone's body, including yours, is unique in how it breaks down and uses food. Then throw in other factors such as your activity level, other health problems, family issues, stress, cultural practices, and such. It'll take a little researching of your own eating habits and digestion patterns placed within the context of your real, everyday world to find out the best way to plan food choices that will keep your glucose levels stable.

Your Glossary of Food Words

Let's start you on your food plan by defining some of the terms you're likely to hear.

Calories. Calories are a way to measure the energy created by the food you eat. So, for example, if you gobble down 1,500 calories in one day, you have eaten enough food to generate 1,500 calories worth of energy. The three major components of food each generate varying amounts of calories. Carbohydrates and protein both create 4 calories for each gram eaten. Fat creates more than twice as much: 9 calories for each gram eaten.

Grams. Food is usually measured in grams. A gram is about 1/25 of an ounce. Looking at it the other way around, an ounce is 28.350 grams. If you count carbs or calculate calories from food labels and lists, knowing about grams can be helpful.

Carbohydrates. Sugars, starches, and fiber from plant sources break down into fuel for the cells in your body and regulate the speed of digestion. Many factors affect how quickly your body digests carbs. Cooking and food processing change the form and structure of carbs, making them smaller and more easily digested. Generally , the more processed the carb, the smaller the particles and the more quickly it's digested, making blood glucose levels rise higher and more quickly. You'll see a bit later why this concept is critical to your food choice success. Most of us eat too many processed carbs and too few less-processed carbs.

Fats. Fats and similar substances come from animal and plant sources. Too much total fat is bad news for your blood vessels and heart. "Good" monounsaturated and saturated fats used in moderate amounts can lower both overall fat levels and "bad" LDL cholesterol levels in your blood, while raising "good" HDL cholesterol levels. Most of us eat too much fat, and too little of that is "good" fat.

Protein. Found in both plant and animal sources, protein is broken apart and recombined by your body in ways that it can use for making hormones, building tissue, and doing many other functions. Most of us eat a lot more protein than we need.

Other food components. Vitamins, minerals, and other nutrients aid body functions. Alcohol is yet another food component. It resembles carbs, but is different enough to be confusing, including containing more calories per gram. Alcohol may help control blood glucose levels if used in *small* amounts.

Moving from Point A to Point B

The first thing you need to do is figure out what you really eat over the course of a week or two. And I mean everything! The best way to do this is to keep a food diary. Write down everything you eat and drink, and estimate the amounts. Don't worry about whether it's right or wrong, embarrassing or bad. That's not the issue. Instead, focus on our goal: to learn more about what you eat and its impact on your health. See the following sample diary. Make lots of copies of this one! You'll want one page for each day. Track your food for one to two weeks, to show your Point A status. Once you've listed everything, then you can assess your current eating patterns.

Now for Point B—where you want to go. How much less should you eat? Let's take another look at the goals you set up in the last chapter.

Your weekly weight-loss goal: _____

Number of fewer calories per week: _____

Number of fewer calories per day: _____

Food Diary	
Date:_____	
Instructions: Under "Meal," list what you have eaten. For "Notes," include relevant information such as whether you exercised before or after the meal, or if the meal was especially large or small.	
Meal	**Notes**
Breakfast:	
Morning snack:	
Lunch:	
Afternoon snack:	
Dinner:	
Evening snack:	
Bedtime:	
Other:	

Strategies to Get to Point B

Whether you want to cut 250 calories, 500 calories, or even 1,000 calories per day, actually doing so can feel overwhelming. What does it mean in terms we can understand? Here are some examples from my kitchen:

- ¼ cup of plain M&Ms has 210 calories (did I mention I'm a chocoholic?).
- 1 gourmet butter pecan, cinnamon, and raisin cookie (no trans fats, but uses butter) contains 130 calories.
- ¼ cup canned corned beef has 120 calories, half of them from fat.
- 1 oat and honey granola bar has 180 calories (no saturated or trans fat, lots of fiber).
- 1 taco-sized corn tortilla has 110 calories.
- 2 tablespoons Caesar salad dressing has 150 calories, 140 of them from fat.
- 1 tablespoon of mayonnaise has 100 calories, all from fat.
- 1 tablespoon of butter has 100 calories, all from fat.

From looking at my list—or your own cupboards—you can guesstimate how much less food you need to eat per day: half a cup's worth of M&Ms, a couple fewer cookies, or the equivalent of five corn tortillas, for example. I think maybe I can handle this! What about you? But if you're having a tough time figuring out how much less to eat, a trip to a dietitian can be a real help. These folks are the pros at knowing the facts of food: calories, carbs, protein, fat, and such.

Choose a Plan, If You Please

So many possibilities: USDA Food Pyramid or the Diabetes Food Pyramid, South Beach or LA, Glycemic Index, Weight Watchers, Exchanges, Carb Counting, Atkins (the company went bankrupt, by the way).... Then throw in conflicting news reports: Caffeine raises blood pressure; caffeine lowers glucose levels. Alcohol has too much sugar in it; alcohol has heart-healthy and glucose-controlling benefits. Sugar is bad; all carbs are the same. Yikes! What's a person with prediabetes to do? After years of exhaustive research, the verdict is in:

There isn't anything you can't eat. Really!

Yep. You read that right. No single food is "off limits" for a person with prediabetes. That doesn't mean it's okay to pig out. But it does mean that you have a lot of flexibility in what you eat—as long as you keep in mind a few principles to help guide you toward the overall healthiest choices. To make your choices easier, you may want to use a specific meal planning technique, such as the ones mentioned above. We're not going to describe all those techniques here—that would take up the whole book. And for most people with prediabetes, you don't necessarily need a complex system of food choices to follow. What you do need to remember can be summed up like this:

- Eat fewer calories overall.
- Eat less bad fat.
- Eat more good fat.
- Choose more "whole" and "fresh" foods and fewer processed carbs.

Assess Your Food Likes and Dislikes

How do you find ways to accomplish these goals? Let's get down to some details. Like the way you identified your personal potholes (stressors), you need to know more about the foods you eat. So grab your food diary. Review it. On the back of one of the pages, list additional foods that you typically eat that aren't in your diary. For each food, consider the following:

- How often do you eat it?
- Why do you like it? Yes, you eat because you're hungry. But there are other reasons, too. For example, I love chocolate. The more stress I'm feeling, the more chocolate I eat. Comfort, economy, routine, ease, habit, sticking with family preferences, and availability—these are other reasons for choosing a particular food. You may come up with even more.
- Is the food a healthy choice? Be honest! If you don't know, check a food list or ask a dietitian.
- What could you do to make the food a better choice? For example, perhaps you should eat this food more often—or less often. You could eat less of it when you do have it. Or you could add ingredients to make it healthier for you.

Beth's Favorite Foods				
Food	How Often I Eat It	Why I Eat It	How Healthy Is It?	Ways to Make It Better
Chocolate	☒ Daily or more ☐ Once a week or more ☐ Once in a while	Love the taste; makes me feel better	☐ More Healthy ☐ In Between ☒ Less Healthy	Choose semi-sweet, limit how often and how much
Nachos	☐ Daily or more ☐ Once a week or more ☒ Once in a while	Quick, tasty, filling	☐ More Healthy ☒ In Between ☐ Less Healthy	Use low-fat cheese, chips from corn, baked, no trans-fats; add fresh salsa and beans

Ready for an example? Look at a few of my favorites in the chart "Beth's Favorite Foods" below.

Now it's your turn. Use the "What You Eat Now" chart. You might need some help to fill in the last column. Ask a dietitian, if you need to. In general, you'll be looking for ways to cut back on overall calories and both saturated and trans fats, as well as ways to add monounsaturated fats, fiber, vitamins, and minerals. To reach these goals, ask yourself these questions:

- Which of the foods you currently eat are okay?
- Which could be okay if you ate them less or made selections that contain healthier ingredients?
- Which foods would be okay if they were prepared differently?
- Are there similar, healthier foods to substitute for foods that aren't that healthy?
- Would you be willing to cut back on how much or how often you eat a favorite food that isn't particularly healthy for you?
- What foods can't you live without? What foods can you cut back on vs. cut out? What foods do you crave or feel deprived of if you give up, leading to a binge?

Beth's Food Rule

Now for those day-to-day food choices. After studying and writing about health and nutrition for years (but remember, I'm a professional writer, not a health care professional), I've concluded that a simple, two-step rule provides most of the guidelines practically anyone needs to make health food choices. Here it is:

Moderation + Variation = Healthy Diet

Okay, so it's not an earth-shattering, world-changing concept. But you can get a lot of mileage out of this little formula. How? Let's start with "moderation."

What You Eat Now

Food	How Often You Eat It	Why You Eat It	How Healthy Is It?	Ways to Make It Better
	☐ Daily or more ☐ Once a week or more ☐ Once in a while		☐ More Healthy ☐ In Between ☐ Less Healthy	
	☐ Daily or more ☐ Once a week or more ☐ Once in a while		☐ More Healthy ☐ In Between ☐ Less Healthy	
	☐ Daily or more ☐ Once a week or more ☐ Once in a while		☐ More Healthy ☐ In Between ☐ Less Healthy	
	☐ Daily or more ☐ Once a week or more ☐ Once in a while		☐ More Healthy ☐ In Between ☐ Less Healthy	

Moderation

I'm a Baptist kid who grew up in a household where the early-20th-century concept of temperance still ruled. Now linked primarily to abstaining from alcohol, "temperance" originally meant "moderation in all things." This concept is an easy-to-remember, powerful guide for eating less. How? Here are some "moderation models":

- When eating out, avoid super-size, grand, big, biggie, giant, king, jumbo, and other "large" words. Once you're used to the "regular" size, you can even downsize further to the "kid" or "junior" version.
- Use a smaller plate.
- At all-you-can-eat places, don't go back for seconds.
- Take a bite to taste, rather than a whole plateful.
- It's okay to leave something on your plate! Remember: You're getting your "money's worth" if you enjoy your meal, NOT if you eat every last bite.
- Serve yourself whenever you can—you're less likely to give yourself too much.

Variation

My concept of moderation came, perhaps, from my religious roots. But variation comes from the adventurous side of me! I grew up in the Midwest on a steady diet of meat, potatoes, and corn. Eventually I got bored and discovered other kinds of food. It's a good thing I did, because food ruts—that is, eating the same things all the time—can lead to several problems that can affect your health. First, when you're not thinking about what you're eating, you often eat too much. Second, you may be depriving yourself of certain critical nutrients if you eat the same things all the time. Variety is quite literally the spice of life. If you've ever wanted to be bold, daring, and adventuresome—

or even if you never wanted to—now's the time to try. Here are a few suggestions:

- Throw in a few spices when you cook. Herbs and spices contain trace amounts of many nutrients, some of which have yet to be discovered. Cinnamon, for example, seems to be the current favorite with some health professionals, as there is some evidence that it lowers blood glucose levels.

- When you're pressed for time and heading to the fast-food place, order something different each time you go.

- Choose one new food item you've never tried before each time you go grocery shopping.

Gaining Support from Professional Food Folks

 I've mentioned dietitians throughout this book. You might want to meet one, even if only for a single visit. Registered dietitians (RDs) have college degrees and have completed internships that prepare them to counsel people about the role of diet in health. Many dietitians specialize in working with people who have diabetes. In addition, many are certified as diabetes educators (CDE). Dietitians can explain the nutritional goals for managing prediabetes, they can assess eating habits and point out areas for change, they can take a look at family recipes and make suggestions for ways to make them healthier, and they can even explain the range of meal-planning techniques and help you choose and try one that best fits your own needs. One dietitian I know, Joan, enjoys taking her patients out grocery shopping to practice what she's preached to them. To locate a dietitian, ask your doctor for a referral, check with your local diabetes center, or contact the American Dietetics Association (see Resources for contact information).

- If your family sticks to a certain type of food as a staple in your diet, look for variations. Take tortillas, for example. White flour and frying are two ways to wreck them, in terms of your health. Try whole wheat, corn, sprouted wheat, or low-carb varieties (usually a combo of whole wheat and soy) at least some of the time, and warm them in the oven or on a hot griddle rather than frying them.

- Check out the natural foods section at the grocery store— or find the nearest "health food" grocery store.

- Go nuts! Nuts and seeds are overlooked sources of mono-unsaturated fats and contain a gazillion vitamins, minerals, fiber, and other lesser-known but still important nutrients. I use ground hazelnuts, for example, as a coating for chicken and fish and to substitute for up to half the white flour in baking recipes.

- Get steamed! Or baked, grilled, barbecued, or broiled, or any other food preparation technique that minimizes the use of fat.

- Go "raw"! True, it's an upscale trend of the rich and famous to eat only raw foods at astronomical prices in chic eateries. But it's also a great idea! Raw fruits and veggies and even some grains are delicious and much more nutritious than their cooked, creamed, canned, or otherwise processed counterparts.

- Explore grains. I just found a yummy grain combo (brown rice, black lentils, and radish seeds) at one of my favorite stores, Trader Joe's. Easy to fix, lots of fiber and other nutrients, goes well with a variety of main dishes. I'd never even heard of black lentils before, let alone eaten them. Then there's quinoa, a grain from the Andes that's a lot like couscous. Speaking of couscous, a quick cracked-wheat side dish, you can buy whole-wheat versions of it at most supermarkets. Then we have beans of all sizes and colors used in Mexican, Italian, Spanish, and other cuisines (plus plain old American baked beans).... It's no wonder the new USDA Food Pyramid people revamped the old guidelines to put more emphasis on these wonder foods.

Overcome Those "Buts"

You may agree that the concepts of moderation and variation are great. And that they can help you implement healthy food choices that fit within any food plan. But.... Yes, there are a lot of "buts," aren't there? And it's precisely these "buts" that can get you, even with the best of intentions. What can you do when you encounter one of these hurdles? Take a look at the next few pages for some ideas.

"My family has certain foods that we always eat—and that I enjoy eating."

- Make a list of your family's traditional foods. Take it to your doctor or dietitian. Have them identify which foods are healthiest, and how you can make the others work better for you.
- Eat unhealthy favorite foods less often, in smaller quantities, or accompanied by healthier side dishes.
- Use similar substitutes—at least now and then. Try multigrain tortillas for flour tortillas, brown and wild rice for white rice.

"I don't do the food preparation."

- Even though you're not at the diabetes diagnosis, check out the American Diabetes Association website or the "diabetes" section at any bookstore. You'll find lots of cookbooks just for folks who haven't cooked much before. Maybe it's time to learn!

- Purchase a book of diabetes-healthy recipes for the person who prepares most of your meals.
- Work with a dietitian to adapt family favorites.
- Offer to help out with cooking whenever you can.
- Have the person who prepares meals in your family meet with a dietitian or health educator. Together, you can make plans to prepare food in ways that will help you steer away from prediabetes back to health.
- Many cooks refuse to change—especially if they don't take seriously your diagnosis of "prediabetes." Don't wait for them to get with the program! Learn to eat around what's cooked, choosing smaller portion sizes and selecting the lower fat and lower calorie dishes served.

"I eat out a lot."

- Order just an appetizer and a side salad.
- Take a diabetes-savvy friend to lunch and review the menu while you eat. Highlight healthy selections for future reference.
- Look for low-fat, less-processed alternatives to burgers and fries. Salads, baked or grilled entrees, fruit, low-fat dairy products, and whole-grain breads and buns are all good choices.

"I'm usually in a hurry and don't have time to put together a huge, home-cooked meal."

- Find "quick recipe" cookbooks for people with diabetes through bookstores or the American Diabetes Association website.

- Try shopping at the deli sections of health food grocery stores. They often have a variety of takeout items that fit within your meal guidelines.

"Believe it or not, I really enjoy fast food."

- Just cut back a little. Once a day instead of twice a day. Once a week instead of twice a week.
- Instead of fries, choose a side salad or fruit (many fast-food restaurants now offer these choices).
- Order water or iced tea with lemon rather than sugary sodas.
- Go for the small or medium version of combo meals rather than the mega-size. Consider kids' meals—you even get a toy!

"I must have dessert after dinner."

- Wait an hour or so after dinner before having dessert. That way you'll know whether you're really hungry for it or not, rather than simply automatically eating it right after dinner as if it were a law.
- Cut back on portion size—say, a two-inch square of cake rather than a huge hunk.
- Purchase or make desserts that are lower in fat. Lots of great low-fat ice creams are on the market. Better yet, try frozen yogurt.
- Share your dessert, especially at a restaurant. Order only one or two for the whole group, and ask for extra forks and spoons. That way, everyone gets a few bites of something different.

"I'm sleepy and starved by the middle of the afternoon."

- Plan on snacks. People who snack have more muscle and less fat and lower cholesterol levels than people who stick to three meals a day! Plus, a steady stream of small amounts of food helps keep glucose levels more even throughout the day.

- Choose snacks that have a little of each: carbs, protein, and fat. Protein digestion uses lots of calories, while fiber makes you feel full. Try whole-grain crackers with peanut butter, an apple and cheese, or cereal and milk.

"I've heard that diabetics can't eat sweets. But I don't think I can do without them."

- You don't have to stop eating sweets. Just don't eat too many of them.
- Eat mini-versions of your favorite candy bars.
- Take one bite, then pass the rest on or stash it for later.
- Use sweets as an occasional reward rather than a daily routine.
- Make your own sweets at home. That way you can control the size and ingredients to ensure that your treats are at least somewhat healthy. For example, I make some mean chocolate chip cookies! But they include no trans fats, plus I put in less sugar than called for in the recipe (and use brown sugar, which contains a few more trace amounts of nutrients than white), fewer chips than called for, and lots of oats and nuts.

"Eating my favorite foods makes me feel better—especially after a stressful day."

- Acknowledge that food serves purposes beyond filling you up. If you feel a drive to reach for a certain comfort food, first ask yourself these "HALT" questions: Am I... Hungry? Angry? Lonely? Tired? What else could you do to address your needs and emotions besides reaching for food?

- Think about other ways you could help yourself feel better—like go for a walk, call a friend to chat, dance to your favorite music.
- Indulge yourself once in a while and don't feel guilty. Just make sure you're accounting for the calories in some other way.

"I'm proud of my heritage and the foods that are important to my culture. I don't want to give them up!"

- Do some historical research. Find out what your ancestors' foods were *really* like a hundred or so years ago. Chances are they were healthier than the versions that have evolved over the years. For example, if your relatives are from the coast of Mexico, grilled seafood tacos using corn tortillas were probably once a mainstay, rather than the deep-fried, battered fish pocketed in white-flour tortillas that are often served now. My friend Lloyd, who grew up in Japan, had a hard time getting used to eating brown rice, not because of the flavor or texture but because in Japan it was called "farmer's rice" and associated with lower-class living standards. Guess what? Even if it was for purely economic reasons, those Japanese farmers had the right idea!
- Focus on other aspects of the foods you're proud of: the preparation, the smell of food as it cooks, the gathering of family and friends, the ritual of passing around the dishes. Celebrate these things, too, and the amount of food you consume becomes less important.
- Identify tasty treats that reflect your heritage but don't also carry a lot of wasted calories. Keep these on hand to snack on and to share with family and friends.

Questions for Consideration

How can you tell if the steps you're taking to lower your calories and make wise food choices are working? After you've made some changes in your eating habits, try tracking your food with a food diary again. Compare both diaries—the one you kept before changing your eating habits and the new one. Ask yourself these questions:

- Are the overall calories you're eating each day closer to your goals?
- Are you achieving moderation and variety?
- Are there fewer foods in your second diary that are outright bad for you?

If you can answer "yes" to one of these questions, then you're making great progress in using food as a way to move back toward good health. The more "yes" answers, the better! Keep up the great work. But if you're not happy with your progress, then perhaps it's time for some outside help. Consider consulting with a dietitian. Check out any of the resources on eating available through the American Diabetes Association. Your goal is to find something that works for *you*, which means finding the best way for you to use your food choices to detour from the path to diabetes and head back onto the road to good health.

11

TIME TO GET MOVING

I can already hear your groan. And I have to agree with you. The concept of "exercise" just plain sucks! The mere thought of going to a gym to tread a mill, like a hamster in a cage, makes me break out in a sweat, and not the good kind. I don't like formal exercise programs—and find it almost impossible to follow that kind of plan. I suspect I'm not alone in this view. But I'll bet there are some activities that you really enjoy. Give me some pretty scenery, a dirt trail, and a good walking partner, for example, and I'll walk—or maybe even jog—forever. Or put on some music with a jazzy beat, and I'll dance in place at the sink while I wash the dishes.

Whether you like it or not, getting physical is a critical part of your plan to get off the Diabetes Expressway. But you should know that exercise doesn't have to be painful or "strainful" to be helpful. You can find ways to work within your health constraints, personal interests, and available time to make "exercise" a part of your daily routine. You'll probably find the benefits are worth it. And you may even start to look forward to it!

The Benefits of Exercise

Too little physical activity helps lead to weight gain. Even more, inactivity may contribute to insulin resistance and higher levels of blood glucose—both things that you're trying to avoid. Muscles store glucose. And when they're inactive, the glucose stays put. Any new glucose made in the meanwhile just keeps circulating around in your blood. On the flip side, regular physical activity—even at a moderate level—provides several benefits. Exercise can:

- Burn calories. Even after you've finished, your body continues to burn calories at a higher rate for a while.
- Help control weight, especially once you're approaching your desired weight. When you burn more calories than you consume, you begin to lose weight. After you have lost excess weight, physical activity helps keep your body burning calories at a regular pace, keeping the excess weight from returning.
- Help increase your cells' sensitivity to insulin. As the muscles move, they use their stored glucose and ask for more. Insulin helps transport the "free" glucose from your blood and lets the glucose enter the cells.
- Lower blood glucose levels. Active muscles need a steady supply of glucose. This keeps glucose moving regularly out of your bloodstream and into those muscle cells. Overall glucose levels remain low and steady.
- Prevent or delay the onset of diabetes. Since physical activity helps your body use glucose more effectively, glucose levels may remain in a healthy range for a longer period of time.

- Lower your blood pressure. Physical activity helps makes your heart and blood vessels stronger. This means your heart doesn't have to pump so hard and your blood vessels remain healthy enough to help move blood around your body. Both factors lead to lower blood pressure.
- Help your body use oxygen more effectively. Regular activity helps all parts of your respiratory and circulatory system work better: your lungs, your heart, your blood vessels. When they are at their peak, your body can more easily and more quickly move oxygen to where it's needed—and remove the "used" oxygen (carbon dioxide) more effectively as well.
- Lower the lipid (fat) levels in your blood. Regular activity helps your body get rid of the "bad" fats and increase the level of "good" fats.

It's not hard to sell the need for exercise. What's the problem, then? Doing it! There are so many reasons we give for not exercising: time, energy, competing demands, other health concerns, personal preferences…. What might help is to take a look at your own situation and determine how you can best increase your own level of activity.

Starting Your Exercise Routine

First off, discuss with your doctor your plan to exercise. Find out what limitations you might have and how you could accommodate them in an exercise program. Once you and your doctor have completed this discussion, then it's time to roll. Or walk. Or get moving in some other way. Your long-term goal is this:

Do moderate physical activity for 30 minutes most days.

That doesn't sound so bad, does it? Here's what I mean:

Moderate: Your heart is beating strongly, but not so fast that you're feeling out of breath or exhausted. Technically, that's between 50 percent and 75 percent of your maximum heart rate. This range is your "target heart rate."

Physical Activity: Formal exercise—or simply anything that gets your heart going and your muscles moving.

30 Minutes: An accumulation of 30 minutes, either all at once or in 10-minute segments.

Most days: Aim for every day, but don't feel you're a failure if you miss a day here and there. If you consistently hit five days a week, you're doing great!

Getting Ready

You can agree with these two statements, right?

- You've already checked with your doctor to find out the range of activities that are okay for you.
- You're not going to start out by setting new world records for running a mile.

Whew! Instead, let's start nice and easy. Low intensity is fine at this point. That means your heart is at less than 50 percent of its maximum rate. You could easily hold a conversation with someone while at this activity level—so if you're out of breath, slow down. If you can do your activity while singing, you're probably not working hard enough (unless your activity *is* singing). You'll work up gradually to the "moderate" goal. Use the following "Target Heart Rates" chart to look up your maximum and target heart rates.

Your doctor may recommend other goals if you take certain types of medication for high blood pressure, which can make your heart beat more slowly.

Target Heart Rates		
Age (years)	Maximum Heart Rate (100%)	Target Heart Rate Zone (50–75%)
20	200 beats per minute	100–150 beats per minute
25	195 beats per minute	98–146 beats per minute
30	190 beats per minute	95–142 beats per minute
35	185 beats per minute	93–138 beats per minute
40	180 beats per minute	90–135 beats per minute
45	175 beats per minute	88–131 beats per minute
50	170 beats per minute	85–127 beats per minute
55	165 beats per minute	83–123 beats per minute
60	160 beats per minute	80–120 beats per minute
65	155 beats per minute	78–116 beats per minute
70	150 beats per minute	75–113 beats per minute

Source: American Heart Association

You'll also need to make sure you've got the right gear for your activity. For any land-based activity, you'll need comfortable, protective shoes. No pounding the pavement in your flip-flops! Look for a good pair of sport shoes with silica gel or air midsoles. Choose socks that can keep your feet dry and prevent blisters. Dress in layers so you can maintain a comfortable temperature during your activity. Have plenty of water on hand— and sip it as you go. Dehydration can mess up both your glucose levels and your heart rate. If you use diabetes medication, ask your doctor about special instructions. You may need to check your blood glucose level and eat some carbs before you exercise.

Get Set

No one says you need to run a marathon or ride a stationary bike staring into a cement-block wall. If those are activities you enjoy, go for it! But don't feel you have to limit your choices to "traditional" exercise. For most people, physical activity should be a combination of activities that accomplish these three goals:

- Build strength.
- Increase endurance.
- Increase your "aerobic capacity" (make your heart and blood vessels work more efficiently).

Some activities may accomplish these three goals all at once. Or you may vary your activities to meet each goal.

But which specific activities should you—and can you—do? The sky's the limit! Let's start by considering activities you might not necessarily find at your local gym: things you enjoyed while growing up. Remember the hours you spent racing around the bases or climbing trees or kicking a ball? Make a list of those childhood activities you enjoyed. Why not try a few of them again? It may seem silly, but these days lots of folks are experiencing the fun of their youth by returning to those favorite activities: softball, kickball, field hockey, swimming, tag, horseback riding, track sports, soccer, water polo, even hide-and-seek.

Maybe you never did any of these sports when you were a kid. Why not start now? Think about activities you always wanted to try but never had the chance. Or consider other activities that get you moving:

- Sports such as boxing or football
- Square or contra dancing at the Senior Center or local community center
- Participating in nature walks at local parks
- Volunteering for the clean-up days at the beach or along the river
- Entering a charity walk-a-thon
- Singing in the church choir or playing an instrument in a band

• Spending time doing a hobby that requires exertion, such as woodworking

And then, there's always walking. It may sound ho-hum, but even a moderate walk around the block adds up to one-fifth of a mile and better health. About 20 city blocks makes a whole mile. Take a look at the "Walk It Off" chart:

Walk It Off	
Miles Per Hour of Level Walking	Calories Burned Per Hour
2	150–240
3	240–360
4	360–420
5	420–480

Walking is so darned good for you that the U.S. government has launched a program to try to encourage every person to walk at least 10,000 steps a day, the equivalent of about 3 miles, depending on how long your stride is. What's the big deal about walking? This simple activity gives your heart and blood vessels a chance to work harder and get stronger. It tones your muscles. It relieves stress.

The wonderful thing about walking is that you can do it just about anywhere or anytime. If you've got an hour for lunch, walk for half of it and use the remaining time to eat and relax. If you've got a dog, a short walk before and after work helps both of you stay healthier and calmer. If you've got a friend close by, use walking time to catch up, vent frustrations, or just share the view. Jane walks with a group of seniors at the mall many mornings, and has found it an effective part of her plan to manage prediabetes, even though she doesn't fall into the "senior" category quite yet. My "personal best" of more than 22,000 steps in a single walk stemmed from an argument with my husband while we were driving. I got out and walked home—not only beating my walking goal but also relieving a lot of stress. If you, too, want to keep track of your steps, you can get an inexpensive pedometer that clips to your waistband or belt and counts those steps. Many health fairs give pedometers away for free.

Then there's what I call "hidden" exercise—moving around whenever you can. It follows a simple principle: *Go for movement over convenience.* Here are some examples of hidden exercise.

- Park farther away from a store than you normally would and give yourself a short walk while taking some deep breaths.
- Walk, rather than drive, to the corner market.
- Do heel or shoulder raises while standing in long lines.
- Tighten abdominal muscles while driving. I use the highway signs for cues, tightening the muscles and pushing my back against the car seat at one sign, holding it until I pass the next.
- Use stairs rather than elevators whenever you can.
- Turn on bouncy music when cleaning the house and dance while dusting, vacuuming, or doing dishes. Thanks to my sister Jayne for this tip!
- Use mechanical kitchen devices or just plain knives to squeeze oranges and chop vegetables rather than electric juicers or food processors. While burning your own energy, you'll build muscle strength and save some electricity.
- Pull weeds, volunteer to mow the lawn, and do other gardening or yard tasks.

- Play with your kids, grandkids, or pets instead of parking everyone in front of the TV like lawn furniture.
- While watching TV or working on the computer, stand and stretch rather than sit and veg. Or sit on one of those large exercise balls to improve balance, gain strength, and focus your energy.
- When grocery shopping, push the cart down every aisle rather than picking your way through the store.

Anything else? I'm sure you can think of even more ways to add movement to your life.

Gaining Support for Your Activity

 The support of others can help make your exercise program pay off even better. How? Take a look at these ideas to see what might work for you:

- Who are the most important people in your life? Sit down with them and explain that you're trying to increase your activity level, and why. Let them know that your goal—30 minutes of physical activity on most days—is a great goal for *everyone* to strive for. Ask them to work with you to accomplish this goal.

- Choose a physical activity that you can enjoy with your spouse, partner, child, or friend. If you brainstorm with these folks, they can probably suggest enjoyable activities that you never even thought of.

- Get a family membership in a gym. Often, family memberships cost only a little more than individual memberships. Make getting physical a family activity. You can all participate in the same activities, all drive together (or power-walk!) to the gym, or all follow your own preferences. The kids can

So what's it going to be? You'll probably enjoy exercise more if you choose a few different activities and rotate them for variety. Plus, each activity gives different parts of your body a different workout, building strength and endurance in all parts of your body. Think of three activities that you'll try to start with.

So, Go!

If you're choosing a formal activity such as walking or riding a bike, you'll do best if you follow four stages:

1. **Warm up your muscles for 5–10 minutes.** This means moving slowly—you could try slow walking or cycling.

take swim lessons, for example, while you do a few laps in the lap pool.

- Sit down with those supporters and come up with a list of ways to add more activity into your day. Once you've created the list, make sure everyone reminds you when the opportunity for adding extra activity arises. It's easy, though, for gentle reminders to turn into nagging, making you defensive and less open to a supporter's suggestions. Give them clear ideas about what kinds of reminders work best for you—and what really turns you off. For example, would you rather have your spouse say, "It's time for you to go to the gym" or "Would you like a ride to the gym?" or some other prompt. If a supporter becomes too persistent in reminding you about physical activity, what can you do? First, acknowledge to yourself and the other person that you do understand they're trying to help. Then identify what it is that makes you sour. Give that supporter alternatives that would work better for you. If you're really fed up, though, simply ask the supporter to restrain from commenting or reminding you about physical activity for a while. Come back to the person later when you've identified a solution that will help better.

Activity Planner/Tracker

Day	Activity	Minutes	Notes
Monday			
Tuesday			
Wednesday			
Thursday			
Friday			
Saturday			
Sunday			

Warming up helps prevent muscle injury and lets your body know that a workout is on its way.

2. **Stretch your muscles for 5–10 minutes.** Ask your doctor for good stretching exercises for the muscles you'll use the most. Stretching helps get muscles ready for action, lowering the chance of injury.

3. **Do it! For 20–30 minutes.** At first you may not be able to do your activity for more than a few minutes. That's okay. If you stick with it, your endurance and strength will grow.

4. **Cool down for 5–10 minutes.** Use the same approach as you did for warming up: slow and easy.

Question for Consideration

Answer one simple question: Are you getting at least 30 minutes of physical activity most days of the week?

If you're not sure, then try tracking your activity with the "Activity Planner/Tracker" chart for a week. Congratulate yourself if you're consistently meeting the 30-minute activity goal. If you're still working at it, don't give up! It takes a while to change old ways. Be sure that you're doing activities you enjoy and that you're finding all the opportunities you can to add "hidden" exercises into your routine.

Once you're consistently more active, you may find that you need to change other areas of your prediabetes travel plan. You may need to eat a little bit more—or less—depending on how your weight's affected by your increasing activity level. If you take diabetes medications, you may be able to reduce them. These changes are signs that your exercise plan is working and that your glucose levels are probably coming down to more normal levels. Way to go!

12

CAN MEDICATION HELP?

You're driving through the southwest desert, admiring Joshua trees, the bountiful range of cacti, the colors of the sand.... You stop at a historical monument and take a look around. In the distance you see a creature running across the desert—a gila monster. What's that got to do with prediabetes? My daughter Mariah, an avid *Ranger Rick Magazine* reader, would tell you, "Spit. Gila monster spit." In fact, the venomous saliva from these lizards contains a chemical that may help control blood glucose levels. The substance is so promising that it's already being tested in people.

Whether it's gila monster saliva, insulin from pigs or other sources, one of the many other types of drugs developed by scientists, vitamins or supplements, or traditional herbal preparations, medications may be an option for people with prediabetes. But what works? What doesn't? And which might be appropriate for you?

Many family practice physicians and even some diabetes specialists may say, "Not yet. Wait until you develop diabetes." However, many diabetes experts now believe that the answer is "yes" when the question is "should people diagnosed with prediabetes get medical therapy?" Why? Several studies have indicated that people whose blood glucose levels are in the "impaired" range may not go on to develop diabetes if they use certain medications. Would you like to know what meds are used? How they work? Whether you should consider using medications? And what about vitamins? Supplements? Herbs? Let's get you the facts so that you know more about your options and what might work for you.

Medications Can Lower Your Risk of Diabetes

When you think of diabetes, you might be thinking of people with the disease who need to give themselves insulin shots once or more a day. That's true for anyone with type 1 diabetes as well as for a growing number of people with type 2. The reason, remember, is that their bodies don't make enough insulin to keep up with all the glucose in their bloodstream. But what about people with prediabetes? One study is in the works that uses a type of insulin to see if it helps prevent diabetes and cardiovascular problems. But most medications used for prediabetes are taken by mouth, not injections. Here's some info about the medications and what they do.

GLUCOSE-LOWERING MEDICATIONS FOR PEOPLE WITH PREDIABETES

Diabetes medications work in one or more of the following ways:
- Help the pancreas release more insulin
- Make cells more sensitive to insulin
- Reduce amount of glucose made by the liver
- Block digestion of carbohydrates or fat
- Substitute for human insulin to lead glucose into cells

Which medications are available? And which might be best for you? You'll need to discuss the appropriate use of medications with your doctor. Some may have side effects, such as weight gain, that may not be worth it for you. Use the chart on page 129 as an information guide (brand names are in parentheses).

Just how effective are these medications? The completed studies showed a reduction in risk of developing diabetes of anywhere between 23 and 56 percent. Note that studies showing the use of diet and exercise had a similar reduction in risk (ranging from 23 to 58 percent). There is also some evidence that medications used to lower blood glucose levels may also lower the levels of "bad" fats in your blood—especially important to you if you have "metabolic syndrome" (see Chapter 7).

The "take-home" message: Don't rely on medications alone to take care of the diabetes problem. But for some people, medications can be an effective part of their plan. Note that many other diabetes medications are on the market, in addition to those listed here; your doctor may suggest one that has an effect similar to that of one on the list. Be sure to discuss the choice so that you feel comfortable taking the medication.

NON-DIABETES MEDICATIONS MIGHT HELP, TOO

Huh? As strange as it might sound, researchers have discovered unexpected glucose-lowering results when studying the effects of medications used to treat conditions other than diabetes. Two of these medications are normally given to lower blood pressure or make the heart work more effectively. One of these meds is used to lower cholesterol levels. Another is a combination often given to replace hormones lost after menopause. As we discussed earlier, there does seem to be a link between glucose levels and fat levels, and heart risk and diabetes risk (review Chapter 7 if you're curious about that link). So it's probably not too surprising that

Diabetes Medications Used to Treat Prediabetes		
Type of Medication	**Names**	**How They Work**
Thiazolidinediones	rosiglitazone (Avandia) + pioglitazone (Actos) +	Makes cells more sensitive to insulin
Biguanides	metformin (Glucophage, glucophage XR) *	Reduces glucose formation by the liver; improves fat and cholesterol control
Alfa-glucosidase inhibitors	acarbose (Precose) *	Blocks digestion of carbohydrates; slows the rise of blood glucose after meals and lowers blood glucose throughout the day
Lipase inhibitors	xenical (Orlistat) *	Blocks digestion and absorption of fat in the intestines; helps lower body weight, glucose levels, blood pressure, and cholesterol levels
D-phenylalinine derivatives	nateglinide (Starlix) +	Helps the pancreas make insulin quickly and for a short time
Insulin analogs	glargine (Lantus) +	A form of synthetic human insulin that transports glucose into cells; works over a long period, requiring only once-daily injections

* *Study is complete and evidence indicates effectiveness in prediabetes.*
+ *Study is not yet completed and results are unknown.*

Non-diabetes Medications with Glucose-lowering Effects		
Type of Medication	Names	How They Work
Angiotensin-converting enzyme (ACE) inhibitor	ramipril (Altace)	Relaxes blood vessel muscles, allowing blood to flow more easily; may stop another body chemical (enzyme) from damaging the heart
Angiotensin receptor blocker (ARB)	losartan (Cozaar)	Causes blood vessels to open wider, lowering blood pressure
Statins	pravastatin (Pravachol)	Lowers cholesterol production, allowing the liver to remove LDLs already in the blood; lowers triglyceride levels; raises HDL levels
Hormone replacement therapy (HRT)	estrogen/progestin (various brands)	Replaces hormones in women who have gone through menopause

medications that help with blood pressure or cholesterol levels also have the effect of lowering blood glucose levels. Which non-diabetes medications seem to help with glucose levels? Above is a list (again, with brand names in parentheses):

With the use of such meds, the reduction in risk of developing diabetes was between 25 and 35 percent. This doesn't mean that you should run to your doc right away and insist on being put on one of these drugs. After all, medications have side effects—some are serious. And these medications can be expensive. It is not known whether other meds within these same categories are effective as well. The bottom line? If you do need treatment for high blood pressure or high cholesterol, talk to your doctor about how you might benefit from one of these medications, both for the condition being treated *and* for your blood glucose levels.

If you're a woman passing through menopause and are considering hormone therapy, the question is more complicated. Many concerns have been raised about the health threats posed by long-term estrogen use. Combining estrogen with progestin may mitigate some of them. You'll need to carefully weigh the benefits and drawbacks of using such a combination. But if you do choose to use the combination HRT, you may be pleased with the results on your blood glucose levels.

And What about Supplements?

Herbal, vitamin, and mineral supplements are readily available in even your local drugstore, with many advertising that they might help control or prevent diabetes. Some doctors say to avoid them, while others say nontraditional therapies *may* have a role in managing your glucose levels. So who's right? Hard to say. The problem is that these therapies usually haven't been tested as carefully as medications. Mostly you have to rely on tradition, anecdotal reports (individual stories), or small studies. Here's what researchers have determined so far about some of these alternatives:

HERBAL THERAPIES

ALOE (*Aloe vera*)
   Benefits: Lower glucose levels
   Efficacy: Seems effective
   Side effects: Side effects minimal, long-term effects
      unknown

AMERICAN GINSENG (*Panax quinquefolius*)

   Benefits: Lower glucose levels

   Efficacy: Seems effective to very effective

   Side effects: Severe side effects, hypoglycemia

BALSAM PEAR, BITTER MELON, KARELA (*Momordica charantia*)

   Benefits: Lower glucose levels

   Efficacy: Seems effective

   Side effects: Gastrointestinal side effects, fever, hypo-
   glycemia, coma

BANABA, CRAPE MYRTLE (*Lagerstromemia indica*)

   Benefits: Lower blood glucose levels

   Efficacy: May be effective; insufficient evidence at this time

   Side effects: Side effects unknown

BRAZILIAN BUTTERFLY TREE (*Bauhinia forficata*)

   Benefits: Lower glucose levels, raise insulin levels

   Efficacy: No effect

   Side effects: No effects on kidney or liver function

CAIAPO, WHITE SWEET POTATO (*Ipomoea*)

   Benefits: Lower glucose levels, improve insulin sensitivity,
   decrease some fat levels

   Efficacy: Seems effective

   Side effects: Moderate gastrointestinal side effects

CINNAMON (*Cinnamomum zeylanicum Blume, Cinnamomum cassia*, and
other species)

   Benefits: Aid digestion of fats, lower blood pressure, lower
   glucose levels

   Efficacy: Seems effective

   Side effects: Mild gastrointestinal side effects, long-term
   effects unknown

FENUGREEK (*Trigonella foenum*)

   Benefits: Lower blood and urine glucose levels, decrease
   insulin levels

Efficacy: Seems very effective; mixed results on insulin levels

Side effects: Gastrointestinal and skin irritation side effects

FIG (*Ficus carica*)

Benefits: Lower glucose levels, decrease need for insulin

Efficacy: Seems effective

Side effects: Bitter. No side effects

GARLIC (*Allium sativum*)

Benefits: Lower glucose, raise insulin levels

Efficacy: No effect

Side effects: No serious side effects

GYMNEMA, GURMAR, MERASINGI, MESHASHRINGI (*Gymnema sylvestre*)

Benefits: Lower glucose levels, increase insulin levels

Efficacy: Seems effective

Side effects: Gastrointestinal side effects, fever, hypo-glycemia, coma

HERBAL COMBINATION (traditional Chinese combination of *Astragalus membranaceus* and *Lonicera japonica*)

Benefits: Lower glucose levels

Efficacy: Seems effective

Side effects: Side effects include diarrhea, dry mouth, dizziness, hypoglycemia

HOLY BASIL (*Ocinum sanctum*)

Benefits: Lower blood and urine glucose levels

Efficacy: Seems very effective

Side effects: No side effects

HYDROPHILIA, NEERAMULLIYA (*Asteracanthus longifolia*)

Benefits: Lower glucose levels

Efficacy: Seems effective

Side effects: No reported side effects

IVY GOURD (*Coccinia indica*)

Benefits: Lower glucose levels

Efficacy: Seems very effective

Side effects: No side effects noted

JACKFRUIT, JACA, NANGKA (*Artocarpus heterophyllus*)

Benefits: Lower glucose levels

Efficacy: Seems effective

Side effects: No side effects reported

MILK THISTLE (*Silymarin*)

Benefits: Lower blood and urine glucose levels, decrease
   need for insulin

Efficacy: May be effective

Side effects: Loose stools, sweating, nausea

**NATIVE AMERICAN HERB COMBINATION (trembling aspen [*Populus
tremuloides*], cow parsnip [*Heracleum lanatum*])**

Benefits: Lower glucose levels, lower levels of fructosamine
   (a form of sugar)

Efficacy: No effect

Side effects: Side effects include minor stomach upset

NOPAL (*Opuntia streptacantha*)

Benefits: Lower glucose levels, increase insulin-sensitivity

Efficacy: Seems very effective

Side effects: No side effects reported

PEDRA HUME CAA (*Myrcia uniflora*)

Benefits: Lower glucose levels, decrease need for insulin

Efficacy: Not effective

Side effects: No side effects

SEMEN PERSICAL DECOCTION (SPDPA, traditional Chinese herbal
combination of rhubarb) (*Semen persical, Ramulus cinnamomum, Radix
glycyrrhizae, Radix scrophulariae, Radix rehmanniae, Radix ophiopogonis,*
and *Radix astragalus*)

Benefits: Lower glucose levels

Efficacy: Slight effect

Side effects: No side effects

TIBETAN MEDICAL HERB COMBINATION (Kyura-6, Aru-18, Yungwa-4, Sugmel-19)

> *Benefits:* Lower glucose levels
>
> *Efficacy:* Seems very effective
>
> *Side effects:* No side effects reported

XIAOKE (traditional Chinese herbal combination)

> *Benefits:* Lower glucose and insulin levels
>
> *Efficacy:* No effect
>
> *Side effects:* No side effects

VITAMIN AND MINERAL SUPPLEMENTS

ALPHA-LIPOIC ACID

> *Benefits:* Increase metabolism of glucose, lower insulin levels, improve insulin sensitivity, lower glucose levels
>
> *Efficacy:* Seems effective
>
> *Side effects:* Gastrointestinal side effects

BRANCHED CHAIN AMINO ACIDS (*leucine, isoleucine, valine*)

> *Benefits:* Lower glucose levels, lower insulin levels
>
> *Efficacy:* No effect
>
> *Side effects:* No side effects

CARNITINE (various forms)

> *Benefits:* Increase use of glucose, increase insulin sensitivity
>
> *Efficacy:* Seems very effective
>
> *Side effects:* No side effects reported

CHROMIUM

> *Benefits:* Lower glucose levels, lower insulin levels, increase insulin sensitivity, decrease weight
>
> *Efficacy:* May be effective
>
> *Side effects:* Kidney problems with high doses, long-term effects unknown

MAGNESIUM

Benefits: Lower glucose levels, improve insulin sensitivity, increase levels of insulin after meals

Efficacy: Mixed results: some show no effect, some show some effect, some are very effective

Side effects: No side effects

NICOTINAMIDE (one form of vitamin B_3)

Benefits: Improve insulin secretion and sensitivity, prevent destruction of insulin-producing cells in pancreas

Efficacy: Mixed results

Side effects: No serious side effects. The other form of vitamin B_3, nicotinic acid, can make glucose levels rise

VANADIUM

Benefits: Lower glucose levels, increase insulin sensitivity

Efficacy: Seems effective

Side effects: Side effects include stomach discomfort, long-term effects unknown

VITAMINS B_6, B_{12}, AND FOLATE

Benefits: Lower homocysteine levels to prevent cardiovascular complications

Efficacy: Effects as yet unknown

Side effects: Overdose can cause nerve damage

VITAMIN E

Benefits: Lower glucose levels

Efficacy: Mixed results: half very effective, half no effect

Side effects: No side effects, no effect on liver and kidney function

You might want to pay special attention to chromium. Although the results discussed here are not clear-cut, many researchers believe that some forms of chromium may be helpful in controlling glucose levels. Several studies are under way to continue assessing it's value to people with high glucose levels.

Building a Medication and Supplement Support Team

 While researchers are slowly accumulating evidence about the value of medications for people with prediabetes, health care professionals may be slow to make the shift in their day-to-day practice. To get a knowledgeable, up-to-date opinion, you may want to consult with a diabetes specialist from time to time. This could be an endocrinologist, a diabetologist, or other physician specialist. Ask your primary care physician for a referral, get friends with prediabetes or diabetes to recommend someone they like, or check with the diabetes center at your local hospital. Usually, you'll meet with the specialist once a year or so to monitor your progress. Most of your care is still provided by your primary physician, who stays in contact with the specialist as needed.

If you're interested in knowing more about supplements that might help, you may want to consult with a pharmacist, a physician who has special expertise in complementary therapies, a dietitian with training in the role of supplements in building health, or an alternative health professional such as an herbalist who works with traditional doctors.

If you're considering the use of vitamins, minerals, supplements, or herbs, be sure to discuss your plan with your doctor. At the very least, make sure your doctor knows which of these alternatives you plan to use. Better yet, have your doctor work with you to integrate any of these options into your overall plan to lower your blood glucose levels. Ask if your health care group has professionals on staff who specialize in "alternative" or "complementary" therapies. And be sure to purchase products from reputable companies. Supplements are NOT closely regulated by the U.S. Food and Drug Administration (FDA). Look for "USP" on the product label, or any other indication that an objective agency has certified the quality of the supplement. You'd be amazed at the strange and even dangerous ingredients researchers have found in many supplements.

Questions for Consideration

If you're using medications or supplements, take a look from time to time at how effective they are in keeping your blood glucose levels under control. Ask yourself these questions:

- Have you given the medication enough time to have an effect? Remember that some meds take a few months to lower glucose levels.
- Are you able to manage any side effects? If side effects bother you, talk to your doctor. You may need to switch meds or change the dosage amount.
- Are you using the medication exactly as prescribed?
- Do you feel better than before you began taking the medications?
- Are you doing everything else you can to ensure that your glucose levels are back within normal ranges? Meds work most effectively when you're following the other parts of your program to control prediabetes, such as losing weight, eating right, and getting enough exercise.
- If your glucose is back to normal ranges, can you take less, or even stop using the medication altogether?

Discuss these questions and your answers with your health care team at each appointment. Find out from them how *they* think the medications are working for you, as well. By following these steps, you'll ensure that the medication is doing its best to help you keep blood glucose levels and prediabetes under control.

13

OTHER ROUTES TO BETTER HEALTH

You've learned about many of the routes to your destination of good health. This chapter focuses on some side trips that might also be helpful, depending on your own circumstances. These are other stops you can make to approach better health and get away from type 2 diabetes.

Get Regular Health Care

You probably do it for your car; do it for yourself, too. Get regular health exams from your primary caregiver, every 10,000 miles (sorry!) or as often as recommended. Your exam should include weight, blood pressure, glucose and lipid (fat) blood tests, a general exam, an exam of your lower legs and feet, a vision and eye health check, and an assessment of your kidney function. Bring a list of all medications and supplements you take, any home blood pressure or glucose results, other records such as food diaries, and pencil and paper to note instructions.

Set Up a Prediabetes Support Team

Have you ever watched a racing competition? A car screaming into the pit, met by a flurry of folks coordinating their efforts to get the car back into the race, can be an impressive sight. You, too, might want to consider assembling a professional support team in your race toward better health. You'll want to check ahead of time to find out if your health insurance will cover treatment for prediabetes (some won't). Here are some health professionals typically available to help with prediabetes:

- Your <u>primary care physician</u>, trained as a medical doctor (MD) or doctor of osteopathy (DO). Their areas of expertise usually span family, general, or internal medicine. Primary care physicians are often considered the "gatekeepers" of the health care system, and you may need to go to one for referrals to other health specialists. Specially trained nurses or physician assistants may also serve as primary care providers.

- <u>Endocrinologists</u> are physicians who have gone on to receive additional training in the body's hormone system. Since prediabetes involves the hormone insulin, an endocrinologist would be well qualified to help with your condition, as either a consultant or a primary care physician.

- <u>Dietitians</u> (RDs) have college degrees and have completed internships to advise people about the relationship between diet and health. Many dietitians have also specialized in working with people who have diabetes and prediabetes.

- <u>Diabetes educators</u> (CDEs) are health professionals who know all about diabetes and have the skills to teach about it. They can help you understand more about prediabetes and what you can do to turn back onto a healthier road.

One of the tests you might have at your periodic checkup is the A1C. This test, also called glycated hemoglobin, measures your average blood glucose levels for the past two or three months. It gives you an idea of how well your body is using glucose overall. There's no preparation for the test. Results are given as a percentage. Anything less than 6 percent is considered normal, 6 to 8 percent is borderline, over 8 percent is high. Your goal is to keep your A1C as close to normal as possible.

- Other health care providers—physician specialists, nurses, therapists, mental health professionals, pharmacists, and other credentialed professionals—can lend their expertise for any special problems you encounter. Consider adding a cardiologist, an eye doctor, a dentist, and others to your pit-stop team as needed.

Monitor Your Glucose at Home

We've talked about glucose levels—they rise and fall throughout the day in response to the food you eat, your level of activity, and other factors. You've learned about the ranges for normal, impaired, and high for both the fasting glucose test and the glucose challenge test. Did you know that *you* can also check your glucose levels at home? Many people with type 2 diabetes check their glucose once a day or more. It helps them keep track of how well they're doing with their plan to manage diabetes, allowing them to discover the daily patterns of glucose and to adjust their plans accordingly. Monitoring glucose is especially helpful for people who use insulin or other diabetes medications. So if you take medication to lower your glucose level, you might want to consider self-monitoring your glucose levels.

If you choose to monitor glucose levels, get used to the term SMBG—that's self-monitoring of blood glucose, the buzzword used by health pros to describe this process. You'll want to schedule an appointment with a diabetes nurse or educator to learn what to do. They'll explain what testing equipment you'll need, and they'll work with you until you can confidently check your own glucose level. You'll need a monitor, a pricking device (most monitors require a drop of blood, usually from a finger), and testing strips. Many monitors store results; fancier models will graph results and download them onto your computer. Most glucose monitoring manufacturers have extensive support and information services, many with interactive websites to track your results.

Start the Heart Part

The connection between glucose and diabetes, fat levels and cardiovascular health, is seemingly tightly intertwined, even if it's not yet entirely understood. If you've been diagnosed with prediabetes, then you're already at higher risk for developing cardiovascular problems. Take your heart health seriously. Make sure you have your blood pressure and cholesterol and fat levels checked often, along with your glucose level. Consider consulting with a cardiologist so that you'll have a comprehensive plan for ensuring your health, with the goal of decreasing your risk for both diabetes and cardiovascular problems.

Keep an Eye Out for Complications

People with type 2 diabetes are at greater risk of many health problems. Because you have prediabetes, your risk may increase as well—especially if you don't do anything now to turn back toward healthier glucose levels. As part of your strategy for staying healthy, be sure to follow these steps:

- Get regular health exams from your primary caregiver. Ask if you need periodic exams from other health professionals.

- See an eye doctor regularly. You might want to have an eye exam soon after you're diagnosed with prediabetes, and then yearly or at whatever intervals your doctor suggests. People with diabetes are much more likely to develop eye problems such as cataracts (clouding of the lens) and retinopathy (problems with the inside lining—the retina—of the eye).

- Check your feet. People with diabetes need to do it every day. You might not need to be so fastidious. However, higher than normal glucose levels can lead to both circulation problems and nerve damage. Your feet are most likely to be affected. So check for sores that don't heal, thickening toenails, and loss of sensation. Make sure your doctor knows about these problems, too.

Identify Your Barriers to Change

I live off a road that crosses a river, one of the few crossings for miles. When winter rains come and the river rises, it's not unusual for the water to flow over the bridge. It's darned inconvenient not to have access over that road until the water level subsides. To warn us about the flooded bridge, the county has a barrier they pull out across the road. One time, I tried to push the barrier out of the way, knowing that the river level was down. No way! That barrier could be moved aside only by a heavy-duty forklift. I was forced to re-route my travel (or rent a forklift).

What barriers might prevent you from proceeding down the road toward health? Let's designate some groups of potential barriers and then take a look at each:

- Your attitudes and beliefs about health
- The people in your life—your "influencers" and "supporters"
- The world around you—your job and your community

We're going to look at each of these barriers, and you'll see a lot of questions, but this time no answers and only a few suggestions. The purpose is to get you to think. Usually, you're so busy with your daily stuff that you probably have little time to reflect on these questions. Now's your chance. You might want to grab a notebook to jot down your thoughts.

Your attitudes and beliefs about health. These attitudes and beliefs are often buried deep down—maybe so deep, you've never even thought about it before. Let's start. When you think of health, what comes to mind? Why? Do you have religious beliefs that influence your view of health? What are they? How do they shape your attitudes? Have events occurred that influ-

Gaining Support from Community Health Workers

 Do you feel like you're traveling in circles, not knowing where to go to get the help and support you need to go farther down the road to good health? Are you part of a group that feels that the traditional health care system just isn't meeting your needs? Perhaps it's time to seek out a community health worker. These people are nonprofessionals in that they're not health care providers. But they are experts—at understanding the community and its needs. A community health worker can be a great resource for linking you up with the services and support you require at this vulnerable time in your life. Look for community health workers at diabetes centers and large health care providers. But you're more likely to find them in unexpected places, like churches and community centers.

enced your attitude about health? Have you dealt with a previous serious or chronic health problem in yourself? In a close family member or friend? What's the role of doctors and other health care providers in your search for good health? How do you view them? As consultants? As teachers? As authorities?

The people in your life—your "influencers" and "supporters." Who are the ten most important people in your entire life? Are they friends, family, acquaintances? Are they still living? Which group of people has more influence over what you do or think? Your friends? Your family? Others, such as experts or authority figures? Of the people who influence you the most, are their cultural backgrounds similar to yours, or different? Have the influential people in your life changed over the years? If so, how? Do you typically agree with the most important people in your life? Disagree? Which of your influencers are also supporters? Will they support you even if you choose a way they don't agree with? Does it depend on something else? What's their motivation for influencing you?

The world around you—your job, your environment, your community. Do you work or go to school? Do you spend a lot of time at home? Alone or with others? Do you enjoy your daily routines? What do you like best? What don't you like? Is your job or major role satisfying? Is it stressful? Is it easy? Is it difficult? Do you feel like you're a part of your community? What community organizations are you involved with? Do you like things to stay the same all the time? What happens when you're faced with a new or unexpected challenge?

So many questions! Take a look at your answers. I'm hoping you'll see some areas in your world that are supportive and helpful in your attempt to travel a healthier road. You might want to circle in green all these positive aspects of your attitudes, people in your life, and the world around you. Now take another look at your answers. What are the challenges or barriers that prevent you from achieving better health? Is it a person's attitude? Your own feelings about health? Something in your world that gets in your way? Circle these barriers in red. And read on to find strategies for turning these barriers into helpers. Here's the formula we'll follow:

Barrier + Change + Time = Helper

Okay, you know some of the barriers. Next comes "change." You have at least three options:

- **Get rid of it.** Remove the barrier from your life. This could be a friend, a particular job, a belief, or any other part of your world that so constrains your ability to deal with prediabetes that you're better off without it.
- **Adapt it.** Change something about the barrier to make it more appropriate to your current health needs. This is a good option when dealing with people who are important to you. You can help them adapt, change something about the situation you find yourself in, or change the way you deal with the situation.
- **Transform it.** Replace the barrier with something else that better meets your health needs. This is often necessary when you're dealing with your own or others' deeply held values, beliefs, or customs that have negative effects on your health. Often the thing itself isn't so bad—it just needs to be directed in a new way so that you'll benefit.

"Huh?" Yeah, I was expecting that reaction. I'll admit that this process requires a lot of self-reflection. But it's an important step if you're going to successfully make the kinds of lasting changes you need to go driving smoothly down that Live Well Boulevard. Let's use Aunt Frieda as an example. She means well, and everyone in the family loves her dearly. But she has taken the concept of the family meal get-togethers to the extreme. If you don't have at least two helpings of everything on the table, she moans and groans and acts offended and scolds you in front of all the others. You've tried simply smiling and politely declining, but it doesn't work. What can you do?

Get rid of her. Maybe you can't ax the aunt. But you can remove yourself from situations where she pushes food at you. Maybe your absence will communicate your seriousness about your desire for better health. Or it may buy you time to become stronger in your ability to resist her pressure to eat a lot. If it's someone other than Aunt Frieda, you may find that you *do* need to cut off the friendship.

Adapt her or the situation. If you tell her what you've learned about prediabetes and the consequences of not changing your ways, perhaps she'll at least grudgingly accommodate your needs. Or adapt your response: Take that helping, but only a bite. Cut back on what you eat the rest of the day to make up for the huge meal. Show up halfway through dinner. Take the extras home. Bring a healthy alternative side dish.

Transform her or the situation. Aunt Frieda or others may face the same health issues as you. Take her to an appointment with you. Volunteer to coordinate a family meal. Suggest get-togethers that don't focus on food. Have a lunch date, with *boquitos* (little snacks), dim sum, or other finger foods, giving more control over what you eat.

The approach you choose depends on the barrier you face. Others' beliefs are hard to change. But perhaps if they see you're serious, they'll at least accommodate your wishes. Maybe they'll change in the future: That's where the "time" factor comes in.

The Next Turn Ahead Is Up to You

You have almost reached the end of this book, but your travels toward better health are still under way. Keep me posted on your progress—and let me know what works for you, either from this book or from other ideas you've implemented.

AFTERWORD:
A P.S. FOR HEALTH CARE PROFESSIONALS

This book is a paper-and-ink version of what I do when I'm having a conversation with someone dealing with prediabetes. I'm not a health professional, but I am a professional communicator and educator. And any time someone finds out I've worked on diabetes materials, the questions, comments, and stories start to fly! So I've come to see my mission as a sort of community health worker in print. My approach is based on my belief that people learn best when they can relate at a more "gut" level to the information. How to accomplish that in a book? Through a personal tone, lots of stories and examples, even some humor here and there, and frequent challenges to the reader to interact with the words on the page through questions, worksheets, and other features that encourage self-reflection.

What about field testing? Accuracy? Documented results? Believe me, I understand these concerns! As an award-winning instructional developer and writer focusing on health care for more than 20 years, a credentialed English teacher, and a member of several professional organizations such as the American

Association of Diabetes Educators, I'm well aware of the need for appropriately developed, results-oriented educational materials. I'm also confronting the realities of a traditional small publisher who doesn't have the resources to roll out a full-scale pharmaceutical-style development and testing program. Frankly, there's a certain amount of "winging it" that has to occur. But it's not a shot in the dark. I rely on many tried and true approaches such as these:

- **What I've seen work** in other diabetes materials as well as in programs developed for persons with other chronic health conditions such as cardiovascular disease, hepatitis C, asthma, and arthritis.

- **A growing body of professional literature** that shows what is effective and what isn't in encouraging health behavior changes.

- **The standards of care** developed by the American Diabetes Association and the American Association of Diabetes Educators.

- **The AADE-7** behavioral outcomes for persons with diabetes and prediabetes. Not familiar with the AADE-7? Look into the American Association of Diabetes Educators website to learn more: www.aadenet.org. I focus on the outcomes that a book and I can support best, such as behaviors highly influenced by personal attitudes, beliefs, and social pressures. I leave most of the more hands-on activities like meal planning and blood glucose monitoring to you, the pros.

- **Prepublication content review** by certified diabetes educators.

- **Ongoing feedback from readers and health professionals** about what works and what doesn't, so that changes can be made in future editions.

I believe you'll find this book helpful to your practice, whether you structure a class or workshop around the book, pass along a copy in your one-on-one meetings, or recommend it as an easy-to-purchase resource for patients who can't afford to pay for formal prediabetes education. My guess is that many of the people who come across this book will never come near your office. Perhaps they'll purchase a copy because they were searching for something about prediabetes online, or because a friend told them about the book, or because they were worried about being given a prediabetes diagnosis and happened to find the book at a bookstore. My goal in all cases is to provide an affordable, accessible avenue through which anyone can learn the basics about prediabetes and what to do about it.

I'll be posting teaching aids, comments from other health professionals, other related materials, and helpful links to my website: www.bethroybal.com. You can send questions or comments to me through the site as well. I look forward to working with you to improve the lives of people at risk for developing type 2 diabetes!

LEARNING THE BUZZ

It seems like the health care world has a trillion terms to describe health problems. In this section, we'll define some of the terms you're likely to hear in relation to prediabetes and diabetes.

Adult-onset diabetes: Another name for type 2 diabetes. No longer used much, since so many younger people are acquiring type 2 diabetes.

Alcohol: One of the components of food, similar to carbohydrate. Alcohol breaks down differently, contains more calories per gram. Alcohol in small amounts may help lower blood glucose levels.

Carbohydrates: These carbon-containing substances originate from plants. Carbohydrates are divided into several groups, usually classified as sugars, starches, cellulose, and gums. Most dietitians classify carbohydrates into three categories: sugar, starch, and fiber. Inside your body, carbohydrates break down into glucose (a sugar used for fuel) and fiber (which helps regulate digestion and absorption of carbs). In general, carbs from fresh, whole, less-processed sources are best for maintaining appropriate weight, steady glucose levels, and optimal nutrition.

Cardiovascular problems: *Cardio-* means "heart" and *vascular* means "blood vessels." Heart and blood vessel problems go together, as the heart is the "machine" that pumps blood through the vessels. A problem anywhere in the system damages how the whole system works. People who have "prediabetes" are *already* at risk of having cardiovascular problems. Progressing on to diabetes increases the risk even more. The reasons are not totally understood; what *is* known is that the same hormone, insulin, that leads glucose into cells for fuel also helps lead fat into other cells for storage. If you don't have enough insulin or if it doesn't work right, the fat continues to circulate in your bloodstream. With too much fat *and* too much glucose floating around, blood vessels can become damaged and clogged. The result is higher blood pressure, clots, and extra strain on the heart. Heart attack, stroke, kidney failure, vision loss, circulation problems, problems with healing, and more are all due to cardiovascular problems.

Cataracts: Clouding of the lenses of the eyes, something that occurs naturally with age and exposure to sunlight; however, the risk of developing cataracts is even greater in people with diabetes.

Cholesterol: A fat-like substance found in meat, eggs, dairy products, and seafood. Cholesterol is used by the body to help waterproof skin, line the nerves, and carry fat around in the blood vessels. "Bad" (LDL) cholesterol can clog blood vessels, while "good" (HDL) cholesterol clears away excess LDLs and fat.

Chronic: An ongoing health condition. Prediabetes and diabetes are considered chronic conditions, for example.

Diabetes: The name given to a group of diseases all featuring an excess level of glucose in the bloodstream.

Diabetes educators (CDEs): Credentialed health professionals who know all about diabetes and have the skills to teach about it. Diabetes educators are often dietitians, nurses, or physicians.

Dietitians (RDs): Credentialed health professionals with college degrees and completed internships. Dietitians advise people about the relationship between diet and health. Many dietitians also specialize in working with people who have diabetes and prediabetes.

Digestion: The process by which the stomach and intestines break down food into smaller particles to be used for various purposes throughout the body. The stomach, intestines, colon, pancreas, liver, and gallbladder are all part of the digestive system.

Endocrinologists: Physicians who have received additional training in the body's hormone system. Endocrinologists are knowledgeable about prediabetes and diabetes, since these conditions involve the hormone insulin.

Fasting glucose test: A blood test to check the level of glucose in the blood after you've gone without food or drink for at least eight hours. This gives an idea of how well your body uses glucose when food isn't readily available. The fasting glucose test is usually the one used to diagnose whether you have prediabetes or diabetes.

Fat: Substances from meat and plant sources that are used throughout the body. Some of the digested fat is used for fuel, while other digested fat is used to insulate your body from cold, cushion important organs, and perform other functions. If you've eaten more fat than your body can use, the body doesn't get rid of the excess. Instead, it circulates through your blood until it can be stored. High levels of blood fat are associated with cardiovascular problems.

Fiber: Stringy, bark-like material from plants, a type of carbohydrate. Inside the body, fiber helps control the speed of digestion, not only of carbohydrates but also of the other components of food. Some kinds of fiber help control appetite as well, absorbing liquid to make you feel full.

Gestational diabetes (GDM) (also called gestational diabetes mellitus): Diabetes that develops while you're pregnant but usually goes away after birth. It's known that certain groups of women are at greater risk of developing gestational diabetes. These include African Americans, Hispanic/Latino Americans, Native Americans, women who are overweight, and women with a family history of diabetes. Problems with pregnancy are more likely in women with GDM. After pregnancy, women who had GDM are more likely to develop diabetes in the future.

Gingivitis: Gum inflammation, often a complication of diabetes.

Glaucoma: Fluid build-up and high pressure inside the eye, which can lead to vision loss if untreated. Glaucoma can be a complication of diabetes.

Glucose: The most common form of carbohydrate-based fuel. All the body's cells use glucose as fuel. Too much glucose in the bloodstream can lead to diabetes and complications associated with that disease.

Glucose challenge test (GCT): A blood test to measure the level of glucose in the blood after you drink a glucose mixture and wait an hour or two. The glucose challenge test may be used to diagnose prediabetes or diabetes.

HDL (high-density lipoprotein) cholesterol: Otherwise known as "good" cholesterol, HDL pulls fat and LDL out of the bloodstream. Having low levels of HDL is a risk factor for cardiovascular disease and metabolic syndrome.

Hormones: Chemicals used by the body to aid in all the body's processes, from making cells to running away from danger. Insulin is a hormone made by the pancreas.

Immune system: Your body's complex system for fending off threats to your health. Involving several organs and many specialized cells, your immune system routinely handles everything from sending germ-killing cells to a scrape on your knee to using specialized chemicals (hormones) to catch and remove foreign substances such as pollen or dust. It's thought that immune system problems may be linked to diabetes, although how they are linked isn't yet well understood. People with immune system problems do have a higher risk of developing diabetes.

Impaired fasting glucose (IFG): A blood glucose result from the fasting glucose test that's higher than normal (signifying prediabetes), although not high enough to be diagnosed as diabetes.

Impaired glucose challenge (IGT): A blood glucose result from the glucose challenge test that's higher than normal (signifying prediabetes), although not high enough to be diagnosed as diabetes.

Insulin: A hormone made by the pancreas that transports glucose and fat into cells. You naturally have changing levels of glucose and insulin throughout the day, to match your body's need—higher levels of both right after a meal, lower levels of both right before your next meal.

Insulin resistance: A condition in which the body is unable to use insulin properly to transport glucose and fat to the cells.

Insulin resistance syndrome: *See* Syndrome X.

Kidneys: Two organs in the lower back of the body that filter out waste products from the blood. With diabetes, the kidneys may become damaged as they tire of constantly removing extra glucose from the blood. Over time, they work less effectively, leading to kidney failure. Kidney problems are a complication of diabetes.

LDL (low-density lipoprotein) cholesterol: Otherwise known as "bad" cholesterol, LDLs often get clumped up and stuck in blood vessels, especially in blood vessels already damaged by high blood pressure or high levels of blood glucose. This makes it harder for blood to circulate easily through your body and causes even more damage and even higher blood pressure.

Metabolic syndrome: *See* Syndrome X.

Minerals: Substances that occur naturally in rocks and soil. Iron, zinc, copper, and calcium are a few examples. Your body uses minerals from the food you eat to assist in a range of functions, from thinking to maintaining your heartbeat. Some minerals are used to form parts of your body, such as calcium for bones. Altogether your body uses more than 20 different minerals.

Nephropathy: Kidney disease, a complication of diabetes.

Neuropathy: Nerve damage, a complication of diabetes. The longer a person has diabetes, the more likely it is they'll develop neuropathy. Nerves are found throughout the body, carrying control signals from the brain to the rest of the body and returning information from parts of the body back to the brain. So people with diabetes may experience nerve-related problems anywhere in the body. Common problems are lack of sensation or feelings of pain or tingling. Systems that are controlled by nerves, such as digestion, may also be affected

Noninsulin-dependent diabetes mellitus (NIDDM): An older term used for type 2 diabetes, no longer used as frequently, since many people with type 2 diabetes eventually need to use insulin.

Pancreas: An organ of the body that manufactures digestive juices for the intestines and insulin to carry fuel from the bloodstream into your cells.

Periodontitis: A disease of the teeth and gums in which the gums pull away from your teeth. The resulting pockets can become infected with bacteria, which thrive on the high levels of glucose in blood. This leads to tooth decay and loss.

Prediabetes: The state in which your blood glucose levels are higher than normal, but not high enough to be diagnosed with type 2 diabetes.

Primary Care Physician: Medical doctor (MD) or doctor of osteopathy (DO) whose area of expertise usually spans family, general, or internal medicine. Primary care physicians are often considered the "gatekeepers" of the health care system, and you may need to go to one for referrals to other health specialists.

Protein: Substances found in meat and plants. Your body uses proteins to build muscle and other tissue, as well as to make hormones and other substances needed by the body. Once you eat a bite of protein, your body starts to disassemble it into various amino acids, then recombines them into the specific amino acids it needs.

Retinopathy: Damaged, leaky blood vessels in the back of the eye. Vision loss may occur. Retinopathy is a complication of diabetes.

Risk factors: Those things that lead to the development of a particular health condition. A link between the risk and the health problem has been noted, yet the reasons for the link aren't always known.

SMBG: Self-monitoring of blood glucose.

Starches: One group of stored carbohydrates from plant sources. Inside the body, starches can be changed into fuel, but more slowly than sugars.

Sugars: The fuels "burned" directly for energy. Sugars come from plant sources. Glucose is the primary sugar fuel used by our bodies.

Syndrome X: The name originally given to a group of risk factors that puts a person at greater risk of developing cardiovascular problems, diabetes, and other health problems. Metabolic Syndrome and Insulin Resistance Syndrome are other names for Syndrome X.

Triglycerides: A type of fat found in the blood. Triglycerides come from the food you eat. In addition, your body can make them from other substances. High levels of triglycerides can block your arteries. It's also known that people with diabetes and prediabetes tend to have higher levels of this fat.

Type 1 diabetes: A type of diabetes in which the pancreas simply stops making insulin. It often occurs after the body attacks the pancreas, mistaking it for a virus, bacteria, or other dangerous threat. Type 1 diabetes also occurs when the pancreas is removed, because of injury, cancer, or another health problem. Other names for type 1 diabetes are insulin-dependent diabetes and juvenile diabetes. Some 5 to 10 percent of people with diabetes have type 1. Without insulin, glucose quickly builds up in the blood. The cells starve. The body begins to burn fat for fuel, creating toxins. The kidneys become overloaded with glucose and toxins. Without added insulin, death would result. Because a diabetic person's pancreas makes no insulin, people with type 1 must inject insulin to survive.

Type 2 diabetes: A type of diabetes in which glucose builds up in the bloodstream even when insulin *is* present. Other names for type 2 diabetes are noninsulin-dependent diabetes (NIDDM) and adult onset diabetes. Some 90 to 95 percent of people with diabetes have this type—about 17 million people in the United States, for example. Many young children and teens are also developing this disease.

Vitamins: Various combinations of the chemicals carbon, oxygen, hydrogen, and nitrogen. Vitamins serve as the assistants or *catalysts* for all the body's functions. Some vitamins help the cells burn glucose, fat, and protein for fuel, for instance. Others help build bone (vitamin D) or repair damaged arteries (vitamins C and E). The list of vitamins—and their roles—is long, and getting longer each year as more vitamin-like substances are discovered.

RESOURCES

The concept of prediabetes is still new and controversial. So it might be difficult to find information about this condition. However, you can locate an incredible wealth of resources concerning diabetes—and most of these resources are appropriate for persons with prediabetes, too. One stop on your route should be the Internet. Almost all the sources listed here have excellent websites in addition to printed information. Whether you're looking for basic information, the latest scientific research, an easy way to track your glucose levels online, or even glucose-lowering recipes, just about anything related to prediabetes can be found via a computer with Internet access and a few clicks of a mouse.

If you don't have a computer or access to the Internet, check out your local public library. Many libraries have computers available for public use—for free. The library staff can show you how to use the computer and search the Internet for a particular topic. Below are some resources that are especially helpful, either via the Internet or by phone or mail. Many of these groups also provide links on their websites to other valuable prediabetes resources.

One caveat about the Internet: Just because you come across some information that is presented in a highly polished format doesn't necessarily mean that the information is reliable. Professional organizations and government-sponsored groups are good places to start. They can link you into reputable pharmaceutical companies, patient groups, and more. Online services such as AOL and Yahoo often provide chat and discussion groups. These are great places to meet folks dealing with the same issues as you. But remember, check out any medical info you come across with your health care team!

General Diabetes Information

American Diabetes Association
www.diabetes.org
1701 North Beauregard Street
Alexandria, VA 22311
800-232-3479 (to join), 800-232-6733 (to order publications)

The ADA is *the* group for diabetes research and education. The ADA provides information, publications, research, and support for people with diabetes. The organization has an extensive selection of guides for all aspects of diabetes, including general information, meal planning, cookbooks, and more. The ADA hosts online bulletin boards (very slow, though, if you're not using a high-speed connection) to help you share concerns and suggestions with other people with diabetes. The ADA publishes several magazines and e-zines for people with diabetes and their families. The group also lists diabetes centers located around the

United States. A free Diabetes EXPO fair sponsored by the ADA also makes the rounds through most major cities in the U.S. Maybe I'll see you there!

Canadian Diabetes Association
www.diabetes.ca
National Life Building
1400-522 University Avenue
Toronto, ON M5G 2R5
800-226-8464 or 416-363-0177, fax: 416-408-7117
E-mail: info@diabetes.ca

This organization provides Canadian citizens with services similar to those the ADA offers U.S. citizens. The CDA has extensive information available online as well as other publications.

National Diabetes Education Program
www.ndep.nih.gov
National Diabetes Education Program
1 Diabetes Way
Bethesda, MD 20814
800-438-5383
E-mail: ndep@info.nih.gov

The NDEP is a joint program of the U.S. Centers for Disease Control and National Institutes of Health. The NDEP provides up-to-date, accurate information about diabetes and how to manage it. Most of the information is relevant to prediabetes as well. You can download publications and view them onscreen or print them out. You can also order copies online or through the toll-free number.

Small Steps, Big Rewards
www.smallstep.gov
U.S. Department of Health and Human Services
200 Independence Avenue, S.W.
Washington, DC 20201

This program created by the U.S. Health and Human Services Department helps people assess their risk for diabetes and gives suggestions for how to prevent diabetes and its complications. You can use their food and activity tracker to monitor your progress. As they say, "the first-ever national diabetes prevention campaign spreads this important message of hope to the millions of Americans with prediabetes."

National Diabetes Information Clearinghouse
www.diabetes.niddk.nih.gov
1 Information Way
Bethesda, MD 20892
800-860-8747 or 301-654-3327
E-mail: ndic@info.niddk.nih.gov

The National Institute of Diabetes and Digestive and Kidney Diseases (part of the U.S. National Institutes of Health) provides a one-stop source of information about diabetes, including new medications that are undergoing clinical trials. The website provides direct access to publications and other information. You can also request publications from the toll-free phone number.

U.S. Centers for Disease Control and Prevention
Diabetes Translation Division
www.cdc.gov/diabetes
CDC Division of Diabetes Translation

P.O. Box 8728

Silver Spring, MD 20910

877-CDC-DIAB (232-3422), fax: 301-562-1050

E-mail: diabetes@cdc.gov

The CDC collects information about all diseases in the U.S., including diabetes. This group takes the research gathered by the CDC and presents it in a way patients can use. They provide a lot of helpful information that goes beyond the stats. They also collaborate with other federal, state, and professional organizations to improve diabetes information, research, and care.

Joslin Diabetes Center

www.joslin.org

1 Joslin Place

Boston, MA 02115

617-732-2440

A large, comprehensive center focusing solely on treatment, research, and education about diabetes, the Joslin Center is affiliated with Harvard Medical School. Other diabetes centers affiliated with the main center are located throughout the United States. Check the website or call to find the Joslin-affiliated center nearest you. Joslin also provides a range of publications about diabetes.

Information on Building Your Health Care Team

American Association of Diabetes Educators

www.diabeteseducator.org

100 West Monroe Street, Suite 400

Chicago, IL 60603

800-338-3633, fax: 312-424-2427

Members of AADE are certified health professionals who provide instruction to patients on how to manage diabetes. The website has a feature to help you connect with a diabetes educator in your area.

American Dietetic Association
www.eatright.org
120 South Riverside Plaza, Suite 2000
Chicago, IL 60606-6995
800-877-1600

This ADA serves as the professional organization for dietitians. The ADA awards the "RD" (registered dietitian) designation to professionals who have completed the certification process. The ADA also provides information about diabetes and diet, and can make referrals to registered dietitians in your area.

REFERENCES

Hundreds of books, articles, Internet resources, and other publications were researched in the development of this book. The
two major sources of this information include:

Clinical Practice Recommendations as published in the American Diabetes Association professional journal *Diabetes Care*,
   volume 27, 2004.
Position Statements from the American Association of Diabetes
   Educators.

These sources are readily available from the two organizations'
websites (*see* Resources). For a complete list of references used in
the development of this workbook, please send your request to
Ulysses Press or e-mail the author.

INDEX

OTHER BOOKS
FROM ULYSSES PRESS

**MANAGING DIABETES YOUR WAY WORKBOOK:
LIVING WITH TYPE 2 DIABETES**
Beth Ann Petro Roybal, $16.95
The first book to provide an at-home program that can be personalized to monitor, track and gain control of type 2 diabetes.

**101 SIMPLE WAYS TO MAKE YOUR HOME & FAMILY
SAFE IN A TOXIC WORLD**
Beth Ann Petro Roybal, $11.95
Sheds light on common toxins found around the house and offers parents straightforward ways to protect themselves and their children.

HEPATITIS C
2nd edition, Beth Ann Petro Roybal, $13.95
Addresses the rapidly changing status of hepatitis C with information on therapeutic strategies and the search for a cure.

FIT IN 15
Steven Stiefel, $14.95
An easy-to-follow, full-body fitness program based on daily 15-minute morning workouts that balance cardio, strength and flexibility.

THE SIMPLE 0-TO-10 G.I. DIET
Azmina Govindji and Nina Puddefoot, $12.95
A no-hassle program to lose weight and maintain a healthy long-term diet based on a simplified version of the Glycemic Index.

STRETCHING FOR 50+: A CUSTOMIZED PROGRAM FOR IMPROVING FLEXIBILITY, AVOIDING INJURY AND ENJOYING AN ACTIVE LIFESTYLE

Dr. Karl Knopf, $13.95

Details how to maintain flexibility, mobility and an active lifestyle by incorporating additional stretching into one's life.

WEIGHT-BEARING WORKOUTS FOR WOMEN: EXERCISES FOR SCULPTING, STRENGTHENING & TONING

Yolande Green, $12.95

Weight training is the fastest, most effective way to lose fat, improve muscle tone and strengthen bones. This workbook shows just how easy it is for women at any age to get started with weights.

WEIGHTS FOR 50+: BUILDING STRENGTH, STAYING HEALTHY AND ENJOYING AN ACTIVE LIFESTYLE

Dr. Karl Knopf, $14.95

Shows how easy it is for a 50+ person to lift weights, stay fit and active, and also guard against osteoporosis, diabetes and heart disease.

FLIP THE SWITCH: 40 ANYTIME, ANYWHERE MEDITATIONS IN 5 MINUTES OR LESS

Eric Harrison, $10.95

Specially designed meditations that fit any situation: idling at a red light, waiting for a computer to restart, or standing in line at the grocery store.

To order these books call 800-377-2542 or 510-601-8301, fax 510-601-8307, e-mail ulysses@ulyssespress.com, or write to Ulysses Press, P.O. Box 3440, Berkeley, CA 94703. All retail orders are shipped free of charge. California residents must include sales tax. Allow two to three weeks for delivery.

ABOUT THE AUTHOR

Beth Ann Petro Roybal, M.A., is an award-winning writer, editor, and instructional designer of health and safety publications, videos, computer-based instruction, and teaching outlines. Her more than 100 publications have been used by well over a million people. She has developed educational materials for physicians, nurses, and other health professionals, as well as for companies that provide health services and products. What she finds most fulfilling, however, is presenting technical medical information in a way that is understandable and meaningful to lay readers, enabling them to be better prepared to take charge of their health. In that vein, she also authored *Managing Diabetes Your Way Workbook*, an at-home program for monitoring type 2 Diabetes. She is a member of the American Association of Diabetes Educators, the Health and Sciences Communications Association, and the American Association of Health Educators.